MOSBY'S
RAPID REFERENCE TO
DIAGNOSTIC &
LABORATORY
TESTS

MOSBY'S
RAPID REFERENCE TO
DIAGNOSTIC & LABORATORY TESTS

Kathleen Deska Pagana, PhD, RN
Professor
Department of Nursing
Lycoming College
Williamsport, Pennsylvania

Timothy James Pagana, MD, FACS, FSSO
Surgical Oncologist
Williamsport, Pennsylvania

Mosby

A *Harcourt Health Sciences Company*
St. Louis   Philadelphia   London   Sydney   Toronto

Mosby

A *Harcourt Health Sciences Company*

Editor-in-Chief: Sally Schrefer
Senior Editor: Loren S. Wilson
Senior Developmental Editor: Brian Dennison
Project Manager: John Rogers
Senior Production Editor: Helen Hudlin
Designer: Kathi Gosche
Manufacturing Supervisor: Linda Ierardi

Composition by Clarinda Company
Printing/binding by R.R. Donnelley & Sons Company

Mosby, Inc.
11830 Westline Industrial Drive
St. Louis, Missouri 63146

ISBN 1-5566-4515-5

00   01   02   03   /   9   8   7   6   5   4   3   2

*With fond memories we respectfully dedicate this book to
Raymond J. Cowden, our "Uncle Ray."*
*In today's world, the presence of a kind, righteous, and pleasant
man represents an oasis to which many are attracted. As a young
man, Ray was honest, kind, intelligent, and competent. His
commitment to his job and his family was paramount. As a
young man and father, he dealt with some very difficult times in
his life in an honorable, dignified, and sustaining manner. In
his latter life, our children knew Ray as a loving, docile, and
caring man. At the end of his life, we remember him to be
distinguished, always in command of his actions and feelings,
and compliant with what life presented him. It is our hope that
his spirit will enlighten the readers of this book to develop these
same qualities and make this world a better place for all who
pass through it.*

Mosby's Rapid Reference to Diagnostic and Laboratory Tests provides the user with an up-to-date reference that allows quick access to clinically relevant information about the most frequently performed laboratory and diagnostic tests. The content of the book is presented in a concise manner in order to allow the user to quickly find key information. Its size permits the book to be easily carried to a clinical service area such as a nursing floor or clinic.

A notable feature of the handbook is its consistent format, which allows for rapid identification of key information required for understanding diagnostic testing. All tests begin on a new page and are listed in alphabetical order by their complete name. The alphabetical format is a serviceable feature of the book; it allows the user to locate tests quickly without having to place tests in an appropriate category or body system. Every feature of the book is geared to provide pertinent information in a sequence that best simulates priorities in the clinical setting. Extensive cross-referencing exists throughout the book. This permits full understanding and helps the user to tie together or locate related studies.

The following information, whenever possible, is provided for each test for effective diagnostic and laboratory testing:

Name of test Tests are listed by their complete name. A complete list of abbreviations and alternate test names follows each main entry.

Type of test This section identifies whether the test is, for example, an x-ray procedure, ultrasound, nuclear scan, blood test, urine test, sputum test, or microscopic examination of tissue. This section helps the reader identify the source of the laboratory specimen or location of the diagnostic procedure.

Normal findings Normal values are listed and, when applicable, are adjusted for age and sex. It is important to realize that normal ranges of laboratory tests vary from institution to institution. We encourage the user to check the normal values at the institution where the test is performed.

Possible critical values These values give an indication of results that are well outside the usual range of normal. These results generally require immediate intervention.

Test explanation This section provides a concise description of each test. This explanation includes fundamental information about the test itself, specific indications for the test, how the test is performed, and what disease or disorder the various results may show.

Contraindications These data are crucial because they alert the user to patients who should not have the test.

Potential complications This section alerts the user to potential problems that will necessitate astute assessments and interventions.

Interfering factors This section delineates factors that can invalidate the test or make the test results unreliable. An important feature of this section is the inclusion of drugs that can interfere with test results.

Procedure and patient care This section emphasizes the role of nurses and other health care providers in diagnostic and laboratory testing by addressing appropriate interventions. For quick access to essential information, this section is divided into *before, during,* and *after* time sequences with each fact bulleted.

> **Before** Important features of this section include requirements such as fasting, obtaining baseline values, and performing bowel preparations. The need for consent is also mentioned here.

> **During** This section gives specific directions for procuring the specimen (e.g., urine and blood studies). An estimate of the approximate amount of a specimen is given; however, this amount may vary from institution to institution. Diagnostic procedures and their variations are described in a numbered, usually step-by-step format.

> **After** This section includes vital information that the nurse or other health care provider should consider or communicate to the patient following the test.

Abnormal findings As the name implies, this section lists the abnormal findings for each study. Increased or decreased values are listed when appropriate.

Notes The blank space at the end of test facilitates customizing the studies according to the institution performing the test. Variations in any area of the test (e.g., patient preparation, test procedure, normal values, postprocedural care) can be noted.

Appendix A presents an alphabetical list of all tests covered in the book. *Appendix B* offers a list of commonly used abbreviations of laboratory and diagnostic tests. *Appendix C* provides a list of typical abbreviations and units of measurement. Finally, a comprehensive index includes the names of all tests and their synonyms and any other relevant terms found within the tests.

We invite comments from users of this book so that we may continue to provide useful and relevant diagnostic and laboratory test information to users of future editions.

Kathleen D. Pagana
Timothy J. Pagana

Contents

abdominal ultrasound (Abdominal sonogram; Echogram; Ultrasound of the kidney, liver, pancreatobiliary system, gallbladder, pancreas, biliary tree)

Type of test Ultrasound

Normal findings Normal abdominal aorta, liver, gallbladder, bile ducts, pancreas, kidneys, ureters, and bladder

Test explanation

Through the use of reflected sound waves, ultrasonography provides accurate visualization of the abdominal aorta, liver, gallbladder, pancreas, bile ducts, kidneys, ureters, and bladder. The *kidney* is ultrasonographically evaluated to diagnose and locate renal cysts, to differentiate renal cysts from solid renal tumors, to demonstrate renal and pelvic calculi, to document hydronephrosis, and to guide a percutaneously inserted needle for cyst aspiration or kidney biopsy. Ultrasound of the urologic tract is also used to detect malformed or ectopic kidneys and perinephric abscesses. Renal transplantation surveillance is possible per ultrasound.

Another use of sonography is in the assessment of the *abdominal aorta* for aneurysmal dilation. Sonographic evidence of an aortic aneurysm greater than 5 cm or any size aneurysm that is documented to be significantly enlarging is an indication for abdominal aorta aneurysm resection. Ultrasound is also an ideal way to evaluate aneurysm patients, before and after surgery. Ultrasound is used in detecting cystic structures of the liver (e.g., benign cysts, hepatic abscesses, dilated hepatic ducts) and solid intrahepatic tumors (primary and metastatic).

The *gallbladder* and *extrahepatic ducts* can be visualized and are examined for evidence of gallstones, polyps, or dilation secondary to obstructive strictures or tumors. The *pancreas* is examined for evidence of tumor, pseudocysts, acute inflammation, chronic inflammation, or pancreatic abscess. Ultrasound of the pancreas is frequently performed serially to document and demonstrate resolution of acute pancreatic inflammatory processes.

Interfering factors

- Barium or gas will distort the sound waves and alter test results. Ultrasound tests should be performed before any x-ray testing with barium.

- The accuracy of ultrasonography is very dependent on the skills of the sonographer (the technician who performs the study).

Procedure and patient care

Before

- Tell the patient that fasting may or may not be required, depending on the organ to be examined. No fasting is required for ultrasonography of the abdominal aorta, kidney, liver, spleen, or pancreas. Fasting, however, is preferred for ultrasound of the gallbladder and biliary tree.

During

- Note the following procedural steps:
  1. The patient is placed on the ultrasonography table in the prone or supine position, depending on the organ to be studied.
  2. A greasy conductive paste is applied to the patient's skin.
  3. A transducer is placed over the skin.
  4. Pictures are taken of the reflections from the organs being studied.
- The test is completed in approximately 20 minutes, usually by an ultrasound technologist, and interpreted by a radiologist.
- Tell the patient that no discomfort is associated with the procedure.

After

- Remove the coupling agent (grease) from the patient's abdomen or back.
- Note that if a biopsy is done, refer to biopsy of the specific organ (e.g., liver or kidney).

Abnormal findings

Kidney

Renal cysts	Perirenal abscess
Renal tumor	Glomerulonephritis
Renal calculi	Pyelonephritis
Hydronephrosis	Perirenal hematoma
Ureteral obstruction	

Gallbladder

Polyps	Gallstone
Tumor	

Liver
Tumor   Cyst
Abscess   Intrahepatic dilated bile ducts

Pancreas
Tumor   Abscess
Cysts   Inflammation
Pseudocysts

Bile ducts
Gallstone   Stricture
Dilation   Tumor

Abdominal aorta
Aneurysm

Abdominal cavity
Ascites   Abscess

notes

AIDS TESTING

AIDS serology (Acquired immunodeficiency syndrome serology, AIDS screen, Human immunodeficiency virus [HIV] antibody test, Western blot test for HIV and antibody, Enzyme-linked immunosorbent assay [ELISA] for HIV and antibody)

lymphocyte immunophenotyping (AIDS T-lymphocyte cell markers, CD4 marker, CD4/CD8 ratio, CD4 percentage)

Type of test   Blood

Normal findings

AIDS serology   No evidence of HIV antigen or antibodies

Lymphocyte immunophenotyping

Cells	Percent	Number of cells/μL
T cells	60-95	800-2500
T helper (CD4) cells	60-75	600-1500
T suppressor (CD8) cells	25-30	300-1000
B cells	4-25	100-450
Natural killer cells	4-30	75-500
CD4/CD8 ratio	>1	

Test explanation

Tests used to detect the antibody to HIV, which is the virus that causes AIDS, were first licensed for the screening of blood and plasma donors. The HIV virus is also known as human T-lymphotrophic virus, type III (HTLV-III), or the lymphadenopathy-associated virus (LAV).

Those at high risk for AIDS include sexually active homosexual and bisexual men and women with multiple partners, IV drug abusers, persons receiving blood products tainted with HIV, and infants exposed to the virus during gestation and delivery.

Because of the medical and social significance of a positive test for HIV antibody, test results must be accurate and their interpretation correct. Therefore the U.S. Public Health Service has emphasized that an individual can only be said to have serologic evidence of HIV infection after an enzyme immunoassay (EIA) screening test is repeatedly reactive and another test, such as Western blot or immunofluorescence assay, validates the results. However, a positive EIA that is not confirmed by Western blot or immunofluorescence should not be considered negative. Repeat testing is required in 3 to 6 months. Until certain clinical criteria are fulfilled, a person with a positive HIV test result does not have AIDS. Enzyme-linked immunosorbent assay (ELISA), which tests for antibodies to HIV in serum or plasma, is the most widely used serologic test for AIDS. It is important to reiterate that ELISA detects *antibodies* to HIV. Because it does not detect viral antigens, it cannot detect infection in its earliest stage, before antibodies are formed. ELISA is used to support the clinical diagnosis of AIDS, to screen blood and blood products, and to test individuals who believe they may be infected with HIV.

The sensitivity (i.e., probability that the test results will be reactive if the specimen is a true positive) of ELISA is approximately 99% for blood from persons infected with HIV for 12 weeks or more. The probability of a false-negative test is remote, except during the first few weeks after infection before detectable antibodies appear.

The specificity (probability that test results will be nonreactive if the specimen is a true negative) of ELISA is approximately 99% when repeated. To increase the specificity of serologic tests further, a supplemental test (most often the Western blot) is done to validate repeatedly reactive ELISA results. The testing sequence of a repeatedly reactive ELISA and a positive Western blot test is highly predictive of HIV infection. Newer tests such as the *p24 antigen capture assay* detect the viral protein p24 in the peripheral blood of HIV-infected individuals, where it exists either as a free antigen or complexed to anti-p24 antibodies. The p24 antigen may be detectable as early as 2 to 6 weeks after infection.

Lymphocyte immunophenotyping is used to detect the progressive depletion of CD4 T lymphocytes, which is associated with an increased likelihood of clinical complications from acquired immunodeficiency syndrome (AIDS). Test results can also indicate if an AIDS patient is at risk for developing opportunistic infections. T lymphocytes are responsible for cellular immunity; CD4 helper cells and CD8 suppressor cells are examples of T lymphocytes. There are three related measurements of CD4 T lymphocytes. The first measurement is the *total CD4 cell count*. The second measurement, the *CD4 percentage*, is a more accurate prognostic marker. The third prognostic marker, which is also more reliable than the total CD4 count, is the *ratio of CD4 cells to CD8 (T-suppressor) cells.*

Progressive depletion of CD4 T lymphocytes is associated with an increased likelihood of clinical complications from AIDS. Therefore CD4 measurement is a prognostic marker that can indicate whether a patient infected with HIV is at risk for developing opportunistic infections. The measurement of CD4 cell levels is used for deciding the initiation of *Pneumocystis carinii* pneumonia prophylaxis and the use of antiviral therapy and for determining the prognosis of patients with human immunodeficiency virus (HIV) infection. As the CD4 cell measurements decrease, the likelihood of a person developing AIDS increases. It is recommended that antiviral therapy be started in patients whose CD4 count is less than 500 to 600 cells/mm^3. *Pneumocystis carinii* pneumonia prophylaxis should start when the CD4 count is less than 200 to 300 cells/mm^3.

The dosage of immunosuppressive medications used after organ transplant is also monitored with the use of lymphocyte phenotyping. Lymphomas and other lymphoproliferative diseases are now classified and treated according to the predominant lymphocyte type identified. In some instances, prognosis of these diseases depends on lymphocyte phenotyping.

Contraindications

- Patients who are not emotionally prepared for the diagnosis or prognosis that the results may indicate

Interfering factors

- False-positive serology results can occur in patients who have autoimmune disease, lymphoproliferative disease, leukemia, lymphoma, syphilis, or alcoholism.
- False-negative serology results can occur in the early incubation stage or end stage of AIDS.
- A recent viral illness can decrease total T lymphocyte counts.
- Nicotine and very strenuous exercise have been shown to decrease lymphocyte counts.
- Steroids can *increase* lymphocyte counts.
- Immunosuppressive drugs will *decrease* lymphocyte counts.

Procedure and patient care

Before

- Tell the patient that no fasting or preparation is required.
- Maintain a nonjudgmental attitude toward the patient's sexual practices.
- Allow the patient ample time to express his or her concerns regarding the results.

During

- Record the time of day when the blood specimen is obtained.
- Observe universal body and blood precautions. Wear gloves when handling blood products from all patients.
- Obtain 10 ml of blood in a large green-top tube (containing sodium heparin).
- Obtain 5 ml of blood in a small purple-top tube (containing ethylenediaminetetraacetic acid).
- Never recap needles. Dispose of needles and syringes required for obtaining the blood specimen in a puncture-proof container designed for this purpose.

After

- Keep the specimen at room temperature. Do not refrigerate.
- Evaluate the specimen within 24 hours.
- Most specimens are sent to a central laboratory. Be sure to draw the blood immediately before the courier's departure to the central laboratory.
- Apply pressure to the venipuncture site.
- Instruct the patient to observe the venipuncture site for infection. Patients with AIDS are immunocompromised and susceptible to infection.
- Encourage patients testing positive to identify their sexual contacts so that they can be informed and tested.
- Inform the patient that subsequent sexual contact will put new partners at high risk for contracting AIDS.
- Provide patient education regarding safe sexual practices.
- Follow the institution's policy regarding test result reporting.
- Do not give results over the telephone. Remember that positive results may have devastating consequences.

Abnormal findings

Serology
AIDS

Lymphocyte immunophenotyping

▲ Increased counts	▼ Decreased counts
Chronic lympho-cytic leukemia	Organ transplant patients
B cell lymphoma	HIV-positive pa-tients
T cell lymphoma	Congenital immuno-deficiency

notes

alanine aminotransferase (ALT, Serum glutamic-pyruvic transaminase [SGPT])

Type of test Blood

Normal findings

Adult/child: 5-35 IU/L or 8-20 U/L (SI units)
Elderly: may be slightly higher than adult
Infant: may be twice as high as adult

Test explanation

ALT is found predominantly in the liver; lesser quantities are found in the kidneys, heart, and skeletal muscle. Generally most ALT elevations are caused by liver disease. Therefore this enzyme is not only sensitive but also quite specific in indicating hepatocellular disease. In hepatocellular disease other than viral hepatitis, the ALT/AST ratio *(DeRitis ratio)* is less than 1. In viral hepatitis, the ratio is greater than 1. This is helpful in the diagnosis of viral hepatitis.

Interfering factors

- Previous IM injections may cause elevated levels.
- Drugs that may cause *increased* ALT levels include acetaminophen, allopurinol, indomethacin, isoniazid (INH), methotrexate, phenothiazines, phenytoin, and toremifene.

Procedure and patient care

Before
- Tell the patient that no fasting is required.

During
- Collect approximately 7 to 10 ml of blood in a red-top tube and send it to the laboratory for analysis.

After
- Apply pressure to the venipuncture site.

Abnormal findings

▲ **Increased levels**

Hepatitis

Hepatic necrosis

Hepatic ischemia

Cirrhosis

Cholestasis

Hepatic tumor

Hepatotoxic drugs

Obstructive jaundice

Severe burns

Trauma to striated muscle

Myositis

Pancreatitis

Myocardial infarction

Infectious mononucleosis

Shock

notes

alkaline phosphatase (ALP)

Type of test Blood

Normal findings
Adult: 30-85 ImU/ml or 42-128 U/L (SI units)
Elderly: slightly higher than adults
Child/adolescent:
    <2 years: 85-235 ImU/ml
    2-8 years: 65-210 ImU/ml
    9-15 years: 60-300 ImU/ml
    16-21 years: 30-200 ImU/ml

Test explanation
Although ALP is found in many tissues, the highest concentrations are found in the liver, biliary tract epithelium, and bone. Enzyme levels of ALP are greatly increased in both extrahepatic and intrahepatic obstructive biliary disease and cirrhosis. Other liver abnormalities such as hepatic tumors, hepatotoxic drugs, and hepatitis cause lesser elevations in ALP levels. Reports have indicated that the most sensitive test to indicate metastatic tumor to the liver is ALP.

Bone is the most frequent extrahepatic source of ALP; new bone growth is associated with elevated ALP levels, which explains why ALP levels are high in adolescents. Pathologic new bone growth occurs with osteoblastic metastatic (e.g., breast, prostate) tumors. Paget's disease, healing fractures, rheumatoid arthritis, hyperparathyroidism, and normal-growing bones are sources of elevated ALP levels as well.

Isoenzymes of ALP are sometimes used to distinguish between liver and bone diseases. The detection of isoenzymes can help differentiate the source of the pathology associated with the elevated total ALP. ALP_1 is from the liver. ALP_2 is from the bone.

Interfering factors
- Recent ingestion of a meal can increase ALP levels.

Procedure and patient care

Before
- Tell the patient that no fasting is usually required. Overnight fasting may be required for isoenzymes.

During

- Collect approximately 7 to 10 ml of blood in a red-top tube.

After

- Apply pressure to the venipuncture site.

Abnormal findings

▲ **Increased levels**
Cirrhosis
Intrahepatic or extrahepatic biliary obstruction
Primary or metastatic liver tumor
Normal pregnancy (third trimester, early postpartum)
Intestinal ischemia or infarction
Metastatic tumor to the bone
Healing fracture
Hyperparathyroidism
Paget's disease
Rheumatoid arthritis
Sarcoidosis
Normal bones of growing children

▼ **Decreased levels**
Hypothyroidism
Malnutrition
Milk-alkali syndrome
Pernicious anemia
Hypophosphatemia
Scurvy (vitamin C deficiency)
Celiac disease
Excess vitamin B ingestion

notes

amniocentesis (Amniotic fluid analysis)

Type of test Fluid analysis

Normal findings
Amniotic fluid volume:

Weeks' gestation	Milliliters
15	450
25	750
30-35	1500
Full term	<1500

Amniotic fluid appearance: clear; pale to straw yellow
L/S ratio: ≥2:1
Bilirubin: <0.2 mg/dl
No chromosomal or genetic abnormalities
Phosphatidylglycerol (PG): positive for PG
Lamellar body count: >30,000
Alpha fetoprotein: 2 μg/ml

Test explanation
Amniocentesis is performed on women to gather information about the fetus. The following can be evaluated by studying the amniotic fluid:

1. **Fetal maturity status,** especially pulmonary maturity (when early delivery is preferred). Fetal maturity is determined by analysis of the amniotic fluid in the following manner:
   a. *Lecithin/sphingomyelin (L/S) ratio.* The L/S ratio is a measure of fetal lung maturity.
   b. *Phosphatidylglycerol (PG).* This is a minor component (about 10%) of lung surfactant phospholipids. However, since PG is almost entirely synthesized by mature lung alveolar cells, it is a good indicator of lung maturity.
   c. *Lamellar body count.* This test to determine fetal maturity is also based on the presence of surfactant. These lamellar bodies represent the storage form of pulmonary surfactant.
2. **Sex of the fetus.**

3. **Genetic and chromosomal aberrations** (such as hemophilia or trisomy 21).
4. **Fetal status affected by Rh isoimmunization.** Mothers with Rh isoimmunization may have a series of amniocentesis procedures during the second half of pregnancy to assess the level of bilirubin pigment in the amniotic fluid. The quantity of bilirubin is used to assess the severity of hemolysis in Rh-sensitized pregnancy. Amniocentesis is usually initiated at 24 to 25 weeks if hemolysis is suspected.
5. **Hereditary metabolic disorders** such as cystic fibrosis.
6. **Anatomic abnormalities** such as neural tube closure defects (myelomeningocele, anencephaly, spina bifida). Increased levels of *alpha-fetoprotein* (AFP) in the amniotic fluid may indicate a neural crest abnormality. Decreased AFP may be associated with increased risk of trisomy 21.
7. **Fetal distress,** detected by meconium staining of the amniotic fluid. This is caused by relaxation of the anal sphincter. Other color changes may also indicate fetal distress. For example, a yellow discoloration may indicate a blood incompatibility. A yellow-brown opaque appearance may indicate intrauterine death. A red color indicates blood contamination either from the mother or the fetus.

The timing of the amniocentesis varies according to the clinical circumstances. With advanced maternal age and if chromosomal or genetic aberrations are suspected, the test should be done early enough to allow a safe abortion. If information on fetal maturity is sought, performing the study during or after the thirty-fifth week of gestation is best.

Contraindications
- Patients with abruptio placentae
- Patients with placenta previa
- Patients with a history of premature labor (before 34 weeks of gestation, unless the patient is receiving antilabor medication)
- Patients with an incompetent cervix

Potential complications
- Miscarriage
- Fetal injury
- Leaking of amniotic fluid
- Infection (amnionitis)
- Abortion

- Premature labor
- Maternal hemorrhage with possible maternal Rh isoimmunization
- Amniotic fluid embolism
- Abruptio placentae
- Inadvertent damage to the bladder or intestines

Interfering factors

- Fetal blood contamination can cause falsely elevated AFP levels.
- Hemolysis of the specimen can alter results.
- Contamination of the specimen with meconium or blood may give inaccurate L/S ratios.

Procedure and patient care

Before

- Obtain an informed consent from the patient and her spouse.
- Tell the patient that no food or fluid is restricted.
- Evaluate the mother's blood pressure and the fetal heart rate.
- Follow instructions regarding emptying the bladder, which depends on gestational age. Before 20 weeks of gestation, the bladder may be kept full to support the uterus. After 20 weeks, the bladder may be emptied to minimize the chance of puncture.
- Note that the placenta is localized by ultrasound before the study to permit selection of a site that will avoid placental puncture.

During

- Place the patient in the supine position.
- Note the following procedural steps:
  1. The skin overlying the chosen site is prepared and is usually anesthetized locally.
  2. A long needle is inserted through the midabdominal wall and directed at an angle toward the middle of the uterine cavity.
  3. A sterile plastic syringe attached.
  4. After 5 to 10 ml of amniotic fluid is withdrawn, the needle is removed.
  5. The specimen is placed in a light-resistant container to prevent breakdown of bilirubin.
  6. The site is covered with an adhesive bandage.

- Note that this procedure takes approximately 20 to 30 minutes.
- Tell the patient that the discomfort associated with amniocentesis is usually described as a mild uterine cramping that occurs when the needle contacts the uterus.

After

- Place the amniotic fluid in a sterile, siliconized glass container and transport it to a special chemistry laboratory for analysis.
- For women who have Rh-negative blood, administer RhoGAM because of the risk of immunization from the fetal blood.
- Assess the fetal heart rate after the test to detect any ill effects related to the procedure. Compare this value with the preprocedural baseline value.
- Observe the puncture site for bleeding or other drainage.
- Instruct the patient to call her physician if she has any fluid loss, bleeding, temperature elevation, abdominal pain or cramping, fetal hyperactivity, or unusual fetal lethargy.

Abnormal findings

Hemolytic disease of the newborn

Rh isoimmunization

Neural tube closure defects (e.g., myelomeningocele, anencephaly, spina bifida)

Abdominal wall closure defects (e.g., gastroschisis, omphalocele)

Sacrococcygeal teratoma

Meconium staining

Immature fetal lungs

Hereditary metabolic disorders (e.g., cystic fibrosis, Tay-Sachs disease, galactosemia)

Genetic or chromosomal aberrations (e.g., sickle cell anemia, thalassemia, Down syndrome)

Sex-linked disorders (e.g., hemophilia)

Polyhydramnios

Oligohydramnios

notes

amylase

Type of test Blood

Normal findings 56-190 IU/L, 80-150 Somogyi units/dl, or 25-125 U/L (SI units). Values may be slightly increased during normal pregnancy and in the elderly.

Possible critical values More than three times the upper limit of normal (depending on the method)

Test explanation

Serum amylase is an easily and rapidly performed test that is most specific for pancreatitis. An abnormal rise in the serum level of amylase occurs within 12 hours of the onset of disease. Because amylase is rapidly cleared by the kidney, serum levels return to normal 48 to 72 hours after the initial insult. Persistent pancreatitis, duct obstruction, or pancreatic duct leak (e.g., pseudocysts) will cause persistent elevated serum amylase levels. Although serum amylase is a sensitive test for pancreatic disorders, it is not specific. Other nonpancreatic diseases (e.g., bowel perforation) can cause elevated amylase levels in the serum. Because salivary glands contain amylase, elevations can be expected in patients with parotiditis (mumps).

Interfering factors

- IV dextrose solutions can cause a false-negative result.
- Serum lipemia fictitiously decreases amylase with the current laboratory methods.
- Drugs that may cause *increased* serum amylase levels include aspirin, corticosteroids, ethyl alcohol, and loop diuretics (e.g., furosemide).

Procedure and patient care

Before
- Tell the patient that no fasting is required.

During
- Collect 5 to 7 ml of venous blood in a red-top tube.

After
- Apply pressure to the venipuncture site.

Abnormal findings

▲ **Increased levels**

Acute pancreatitis

Penetrating peptic
  ulcer

Perforated peptic ulcer

Necrotic bowel

Perforated bowel

Acute cholecystitis

Parotiditis (mumps)

Ectopic pregnancy

Pulmonary infarction

Diabetic ketoacidosis

Chronic relapsing pancreatitis

Duodenal obstruction

notes

antinuclear antibody (ANA)

Type of test Blood

Normal findings No ANA detected in a titer with a dilution
>1:20

Test explanation

ANA is a group of antinuclear antibodies used to diagnose systemic lupus erythematosus (SLE). Because almost all patients
with SLE develop autoantibodies, a negative ANA test excludes
the diagnosis. Positive results occur in approximately 95% of patients with this disease; however, many other rheumatic diseases
are also associated with ANA.

There are several different patterns of fluorescence, seen by the
UV microscope. When combined with the specific subtype of
ANA, the pattern can increase specificity of the ANA subtypes for
the various autoimmune diseases. As the diseases become less active because of therapy, the ANA titers can be expected to fall.
None of the ANA subtypes are exclusive for any one autoimmune
disease.

Interfering factors

✠ Drugs that may cause a *false-positive* ANA test include chlo-
rothiazides, griseofulvin, hydralazine, penicillin, phenytoin
sodium, procainamide, and sulfonamides.

Procedure and patient care

Before

- Tell the patient that no fasting or preparation is required.

During

- Collect 7 to 10 ml of venous blood in a red-top tube.
- Indicate on the laboratory slip any drugs that may affect the
  test results.

After

- Apply pressure to the venipuncture site.

Abnormal findings

▲ **Increased levels**

SLE
Rheumatoid arthritis
Chronic hepatitis
Periarteritis (polyarteritis) nodosa
Dermatomyositis
Scleroderma
Infectious mononucleosis
Raynaud's disease
Sjögren syndrome
Other immune diseases
Leukemia
Myasthenia gravis
Cirrhosis

notes

arterial blood gases (Blood gases [ABGs])

Type of test Blood

Normal findings

pH
Adult/child: 7.35-7.45
Newborn: 7.32-7.49
2 months-2 years: 7.34-7.46
pH (venous) 7.31-7.41

Pco_2
Adult/child: 35-45 mm Hg
Child <2 years: 26-41 mm Hg
Pco_2 (venous) 40-50 mm Hg

HCO_3^-
Adult/child: 21-28 mEq/L
Newborn/infant: 16-24 mEq/L

Po_2
Adult/child: 80-100 mm Hg
Newborn: 60-70 mm Hg
Po_2 (venous) 40-50 mm Hg

O_2 saturation
Adult/child: 95% to 100%
Elderly: 95%
Newborn: 40% to 90%
O_2 content (arterial) 15-22 vol %
O_2 content (venous) 11-16 vol %

Possible critical values

pH: <7.25 or >7.55
Pco_2: <20 or >60
HCO_3^-: <15 or >40
Po_2: <40
O_2 saturation: 75% or lower
Base Excess: ±3 mEq/L

Test explanation

Measurement of ABGs provides valuable information in assessing and managing a patient's respiratory (ventilation) and metabolic (renal) acid/base and electrolyte homeostasis. It is also used to assess adequacy of oxygenation. ABGs are used to monitor patients on ventilators, monitor critically ill nonventilator patients, establish preoperative baseline parameters, and enlighten electrolyte therapy.

pH

The pH is inversely proportional to the actual hydrogen ion concentration. Therefore, as the hydrogen ion concentration decreases, the pH increases, and vice versa. In respiratory or metabolic alkalosis, the pH is elevated; in respiratory or metabolic acidosis, the pH is decreased.

P_{CO_2}

The P_{CO_2} is a measure of the partial pressure of CO_2 in the blood. P_{CO_2} is a measurement of ventilation capability. The faster and more deeply one breathes, the more CO_2 is blown off, and P_{CO_2} levels drop. The P_{CO_2} level and the pH are inversely proportional. The P_{CO_2} in the blood and cerebrospinal fluid is a major stimulant to the breathing center in the brain. As P_{CO_2} levels rise, breathing is stimulated. The P_{CO_2} level is elevated in primary respiratory acidosis and decreased in primary respiratory alkalosis. Because the lungs compensate for primary metabolic acid-base derangements, P_{CO_2} levels are affected by metabolic disturbances as well. In metabolic acidosis, the lungs attempt to compensate by "blowing off" CO_2 to raise pH. In metabolic alkalosis, the lungs attempt to compensate by retaining CO_2 to lower pH.

Bicarbonate (HCO_3^-) or CO_2 content

Most of the CO_2 content in the blood is HCO_3^-. The bicarbonate ion is a measure of the *metabolic (renal/kidney)* component of acid-base equilibrium. It is regulated by the kidney. This ion can be measured directly by the bicarbonate value or indirectly by the CO_2 content (see p. 66). The relationship of bicarbonate to pH is directly proportional. HCO_3^- is elevated in metabolic alkalosis and decreased in metabolic acidosis. The kidneys also are used to compensate for primary respiratory acid-base derangements. For example, in respiratory acidosis, the kidneys attempt to compensate by resorbing increased amounts of HCO_3^-. In respiratory alkalosis, the kidneys excrete HCO_3^- in increased amounts in an attempt to lower pH through compensation.

Po$_2$

Po$_2$ is a measure of the tension (pressure) of oxygen dissolved in the plasma. This pressure determines the force of O_2 to diffuse across the pulmonary alveoli membrane. The Po$_2$ level is decreased in:

1. Patients who are unable to oxygenate the arterial blood because of O_2 diffusion difficulties (e.g., pneumonia, shock lung, congestive failure)
2. Patients who have premature mixing of venous blood with arterial blood (e.g., in congenital heart disease)
3. Patients who have underventilated and overperfused pulmonary alveoli (Pickwickian syndrome [i.e., obese patients who cannot breathe properly when in the supine position or patients with significant atelectasis])

O$_2$ saturation

Oxygen saturation is an indication of the percentage of hemoglobin saturated with O_2. When 92% to 100% of the hemoglobin carries O_2, the tissues are adequately provided with O_2, assuming normal O_2 dissociation. Pulse oximetry (see p. 206) is a noninvasive method of determining O_2 saturation. This can be done easily and continuously.

Base excess/deficit

This number represents the amount of buffering anions in the blood. Negative base excess (deficit) indicates a metabolic acidosis (e.g., lactic acidosis). A positive base excess indicates metabolic alkalosis or compensation to prolonged respiratory acidosis.

Contraindications

- Negative Allen's test indicating that there is no ulnar artery
- AV fistula proximal to the site of proposed access
- Severe coagulopathy

Potential complications

- Occlusion of the artery used for access
- Penetration of other important structures anatomically juxtaposed to the artery (e.g., nerve)

Interfering factors

- O_2 saturation can be falsely increased with the inhalation of carbon monoxide.
- Respiration can be inhibited by the use of sedative hypnotics or narcotics.

Procedure and patient care

Before

- Notify the laboratory before drawing ABGs so that the necessary equipment can be calibrated before the blood sample arrives.
- Perform the Allen test to assess collateral circulation.

During

- Note that arterial blood can be obtained from any area of the body where strong pulses are palpable, usually from the radial, brachial, or femoral artery.
- Cleanse the arterial site.
- Consider applying 0.5 ml of lidocaine in the skin overlying the proposed access site.
- Attach a 20-gauge needle to a syringe containing approximately 0.2 ml of heparin. After drawing 3 to 5 ml of blood, remove the needle and apply pressure to the arterial site for 3 to 5 minutes.
- Expel any air bubbles in the syringe.
- Cap the syringe and gently rotate to mix the blood and heparin.
- Indicate on the laboratory slip if the patient is receiving oxygen therapy or is attached to a ventilator.
- Note that an arterial puncture is performed by laboratory technicians, respiratory-inhalation therapists, nurses, or physicians in approximately 10 minutes.
- Tell the patient that the arterial puncture is associated with more discomfort than a venous puncture.

After

- Place the arterial blood on ice and immediately take it to the chemistry laboratory for analysis.
- Apply pressure or a pressure dressing to the arterial puncture site for 3 to 5 minutes to avoid hematoma formation.
- Assess the puncture site for bleeding. Remember that an artery rather than a vein has been stuck.
- If the patient has an abnormal clotting time or is taking anticoagulants, apply pressure for a longer period (approximately 15 minutes).

Abnormal findings

▲ **Increased pH (alkalosis)**

Metabolic alkalosis
Hypokalemia
Hypochloremia
Chronic and high volume
  gastric suction
Chronic vomiting
Aldosteronism
Mercurial diuretics
Respiratory alkalosis
Chronic heart failure
Cystic fibrosis
Carbon monoxide poi-
  soning
Pulmonary emboli
Shock
Acute severe pulmonary
  diseases
Anxiety neuroses
Pain
Pregnancy

▼ **Decreased pH (acidosis)**

Metabolic acidosis
Ketoacidosis
Lactic acidosis
Severe diarrhea
Renal failure
Respiratory acidosis
Respiratory failure

▲ **Increased P_{CO_2}**

Chronic obstructive pul-
  monary disease (COPD)
  (bronchitis, emphysema)
Oversedation
Head trauma
Overoxygenation in a
  patient with COPD
Pickwickian syndrome

▼ **Decreased P_{CO_2}**

Hypoxemia
Pulmonary emboli
Anxiety
Pain
Pregnancy

▲ **Increased P_{O_2}, increased O_2 content**
Polycythemia
Increased inspired O_2
Hyperventilation

▼ **Decreased P_{O_2}, decreased O_2 content**
Anemias
Mucus plug
Bronchospasm
Atelectasis
Pneumothorax
Pulmonary edema
Adult respiratory distress syndrome
Restrictive lung disease
Atrial or ventricular cardiac septal defects
Emboli
Inadequate O_2 in inspired air (suffocation)
Severe hypoventilation (e.g., oversedation, neurologic somnolence)

▲ **Increased HCO_3^-**
Chronic vomiting
Chronic high volume gastric suction
Aldosteronism
Use of mercurial diuretics
COPD

▼ **Decreased HCO_3^-**
Chronic and severe diarrhea
Chronic use of loop diuretics
Starvation
Diabetic ketoacidosis
Acute renal failure

notes

arteriography (Angiography)

Type of test X-ray with contrast dye

Normal findings Normal arterial vasculature

Test explanation

With the injection of radioopaque contrast material into arteries, blood vessels can be visualized to determine arterial anatomy, vascular disease, or neoplasms. With a catheter usually placed through the femoral artery and into the desired artery, radioopaque contrast is rapidly injected while x-ray films are obtained. Blood flow dynamics, abnormal blood vessels, vascular anomalies, normal and abnormal vascular anatomy, and tumors are easily seen.

Digital subtraction angiography is a sophisticated type of computerized fluoroscopy that, when used with arterial angiography, can better visualize the arteries of the body, especially the carotid and cerebral arteries. It is especially useful when adjacent bone inhibits visualization of the blood vessel to be evaluated.

Although nearly all major blood vessels can be visualized through the technique of arteriography, the kidneys, adrenal glands, brain, and abdominal aorta (with lower extremities) are most usually visualized.

Renal angiography permits evaluation of blood flow dynamics, demonstration of abnormal blood vessels, and differentiation of avascular renal cyst from hypervascular renal cancers. Arteriosclerotic narrowing (stenosis) of the renal artery is best demonstrated with this study. The angiographic location of the stenotic area is helpful for the vascular surgeon considering repair. Complete transection of the renal artery by blunt or penetrating trauma can also be seen as total vascular obstruction. Highly vascular renal cancers can produce a "blush" of contrast material during angiography.

Cerebral angiography provides radiographic visualization of the cerebral vascular system with the injection of radioopaque dye into the carotid or vertebral arteries. With this procedure, abnormalities of the cerebral circulation such as aneurysms, occlusions, stenosis, or arteriovenous (AV) malformations can be identified. A vascular tumor is seen as a mass containing small, abnormal blood vessels. A nonvascular tumor, abscess, or hematoma appears as a mass distorting the normal vascular contour.

Lower extremity arteriography allows for accurate identification and location of occlusions within the abdominal aorta and lower extremity arteries. Total or near-total occlusion of the flow of dye is seen in arteriosclerotic vascular occlusive disease. Emboli are seen as total occlusions of the artery. Arterial traumas such as lacerations or intimal tears (laceration of the arterial inner lining) likewise appear as total or near-total obstruction of the flow of dye. Aneurysmal dilation of the arteries or its branches also can be seen. Unusual arterial disorders such as Buerger's disease and fibromuscular dysplasia have the classic arterial "beading," which is pathognomonic.

Arterial vascular balloon dilation can be performed if a short segment arterial stenosis is identified.

Contraindications

- Patients with allergies to shellfish or iodinated dye
- Patients who are uncooperative or agitated
- Patients who are pregnant
- Patients with renal disorders, because iodinated contrast is nephrotoxic
- Patients with a bleeding propensity
- Patients who are dehydrated, because they are especially susceptible to dye-induced renal failure

Potential complications

- Allergic reaction to iodinated dye
- Hemorrhage from the arterial puncture site used for arterial access
- Arterial embolism from dislodgment of an arteriosclerotic plaque
- Soft tissue infection around the puncture site
- Renal failure, especially in elderly patients who are chronically dehydrated or have a mild degree of renal failure
- Dissection of the intimal lining of the artery causing complete or partial arterial occlusion
- Pseudoaneurysm development as a result of failure of the puncture site to seal
- Hypoglycemia or acidosis in patients who are taking metformin (Glucophage) and receive iodine dye

Procedure and patient care

A

Before

- Explain the procedure to the patient. Allay any fears and allow the patient to verbalize concerns.
- Ensure that written and informed consent for this procedure is in the patient's chart.
- Inform the patient that a warm flush may be felt when the dye is injected.
- Assess the possibility of allergies to iodinated dye.
- Determine if the patient has been taking anticoagulants.
- Keep the patient NPO for at least 2 to 8 hours before testing.
- Mark the site of the patient's peripheral pulses with a pen before arterial catheterization. This will permit assessment of the peripheral pulses after the procedure.
- Administer preprocedural medications as ordered.
- For cerebral angiograms, perform a baseline neurologic assessment to compare subsequent assessments. This is to potentially diagnose any strokes that may be precipitated by cerebral arteriography.
- Instruct the patient to void before the study because the iodinated dye can act as an osmotic diuretic.

During

- The femoral artery is cannulated, and a wire is threaded up that artery and into or near the opening of the desired artery to be examined.
- A catheter is then placed over that wire. The wire is removed.
- Through the catheter, iodinated contrast material is injected by the use of an automated injector at a preset, controlled rate. This occurs over several seconds.
- Serial x-ray films are taken in timed sequence to show the arterial injection, and subsequent x-ray films are taken to show the venous phase of the injection.
- Note that this procedure is usually performed by an angiographer (radiologist) in approximately 1 to 2 hours.
- During the dye injection, remind the patient that an intense, burning flush may be felt throughout the body but lasts only a few seconds.

After

- X-ray studies are completed, the catheter is removed, and a pressure dressing is applied to the puncture site.
- Monitor the patient's vital signs for indications of hemorrhage.
- Assess the peripheral arterial pulse in the extremity used for vascular access and compare it with the preprocedural baseline values.
- Perform a neurologic assessment for any signs of catheter-induced embolic stroke syndrome if cerebral arteriography is performed.
- Observe the arterial puncture site frequently for signs of bleeding or hematoma.
- Maintain pressure at the puncture site with a 1- to 2-pound sandbag or an IV bag.
- Keep the patient on bed rest for about 8 hours following the procedure to allow for complete sealing of the arterial puncture site.
- Assess the patient's extremities for signs of loss of blood supply (e.g., loss of pulses, numbness, pallor, tingling, pain, loss of sensory/motor function).
- Note and compare the color and temperature of the extremity with that of the uninvolved extremity.
- Administer mild analgesics for minor discomfort at the arterial puncture site.
- Have the patient drink fluids to prevent dehydration caused by the diuretic action of the dye.

Abnormal findings

Arteriography of the lower extremity

Arteriosclerotic occlusion
Embolus occlusion
Primary arterial diseases (e.g., fibromuscular dysplasia, Buerger's disease)

Aneurysm
Aberrant arterial anatomy
Tumor neovascularity
Neoplastic arterial compression

Brain arteriography

Vascular aneurysm	Abscess
Vascular occlusion or stenosis	Hematoma
Vascular AV malformations	Cerebral vascular thrombosis
Tumor	

Kidney arteriography

Anatomic aberrant blood vessels	Arthrosclerotic narrowing of the renal artery
Renal cyst	Renal vascular causes of hypertension
Renal solid tumor	

notes

arthroscopy

Type of test Endoscopy

Normal findings Normal ligaments, menisci, and articular surfaces of the joint

Test explanation

Arthroscopy is an endoscopic procedure that allows examination of a joint interior with a specially designed endoscope. Although this technique can visualize many joints of the body, it is most often used to evaluate the knee for meniscus cartilage or ligament injury. It is also used in the differential diagnosis of acute and chronic disorders of the knee (e.g., arthritic inflammation vs. injury).

Physicians can now perform corrective surgery on the knee through the endoscope. Meniscus removal, spur removal, ligamentous repair, and biopsy are but a few of the procedures that are done through the arthroscope. Because a large incision is avoided, recovery is faster and more comfortable.

Arthroscopy is also used to monitor the progression of disease and the effectiveness of therapy. Joints that can be evaluated by the arthroscope include the tarsal, ankle, knee, hip, carpal, wrist, shoulder, and temporomandibular joints.

Contraindications

- Patients with ankylosis
- Patients with local skin or wound infections

Potential complications

- Infection
- Hemarthrosis
- Swelling
- Joint injury
- Synovial rupture

Procedure and patient care

Before

- Explain the procedure to the patient.
- Ensure that the physician has obtained written consent for this procedure.
- Keep the patient NPO after midnight on the day of the test.

- Instruct the patient who will use crutches after the procedure regarding the appropriate crutch gait. The patient should use crutches after arthroscopy until he or she can walk without limping.
- Shave the hair in the area 6 inches above and below the joint before the test (as ordered).

During

- Place the patient on his or her back on an operating room table.
- Local or general anesthesia is used.
- A small incision is made in the skin around the knee.
- The arthroscope (a lighted instrument) is inserted into the joint space to visualize the inside of the knee joint.
- Afterwards a few stitches are placed into the skin, and a pressure dressing is applied over the incision site.
- Note that this procedure is performed in the operating room by an orthopedic surgeon in approximately 15 to 30 minutes.

After

- Instruct the patient to elevate the knee when sitting and to avoid overbending the knee so that swelling is minimized.
- Inform the patient that he or she can usually walk with the assistance of crutches; however, this depends on the extent of the procedure and the physician's protocol.
- Tell the patient to minimize use of the joint for several days.
- Apply ice to reduce pain and swelling.

Abnormal findings

Torn cartilage

Torn ligament

Patellar disease

Patellar fracture

Chondromalacia

Osteochondritis dissecans

Cyst (e.g., Baker's)

Synovitis

Osteoarthritis

Rheumatoid arthritis

Degenerative arthritis

Meniscal disease

Osteochondromatosis

Trapped synovium

notes

aspartate aminotransferase (AST; formerly called Serum glutamic-oxaloacetic transaminase [SGOT])

Type of test Blood

Normal findings

Adult: 8-20 U/L, 5-40 IU/L, or 8-20 U/L (SI units);
    females tend to have slightly lower values than males
Elderly: values slightly higher than adult
Child: values similar to adult
Newborn/infant: 15-60 U/L

Test explanation

This test is used in the evaluation of suspected coronary occlusive heart disease or suspected hepatocellular diseases. Serum AST levels become elevated 8 hours after cell injury, peak at 24 to 36 hours, and return to normal in 3 to 7 days. If the cellular injury is chronic, levels will be persistently elevated.

AST was formerly known as *SGOT*. The AST/SGOT enzyme is one of the enzymes tested in the cardiac enzyme series. Although not specific for myocardial injury, when observed with the enzymes creatine phosphokinase (CPK, see p. 95) and lactate dehydrogenase (LDH, see p. 173), it is useful in diagnosis of a myocardial infarction (MI). Myocardial injuries such as angina, pericarditis, or rheumatic carditis do not increase the AST level.

Because AST also exists within the liver cells, diseases that affect the hepatocyte cause elevated levels of this enzyme. In acute hepatitis, AST levels can rise 20 times the normal value. In acute extrahepatic obstruction (e.g., gallstone), AST levels quickly rise to 10 times the normal and swiftly fall.

Serum AST levels are often compared with alanine aminotransferase (ALT, see p. 9) levels. The AST/ALT ratio is usually greater than 1.0 in patients with alcoholic cirrhosis, liver congestion, and metastatic tumor of the liver. Ratios less than 1.0 may be seen in patients with acute hepatitis, viral hepatitis, or infectious mononucleosis. The ratio is less accurate if AST levels exceed 10 times normal.

Patients with acute pancreatitis, acute renal diseases, musculoskeletal diseases, or trauma may have a transient rise in serum AST. Patients with red blood cell abnormalities such as acute hemolytic anemia and severe burns also can have elevations of this enzyme.

Interfering factors

- Exercise may cause increased levels.
- Drugs that may cause *increased* levels include antihypertensives, cholinergic agents, coumarin-type anticoagulants, digitalis preparations, erythromycin, isoniazid, oral contraceptives, salicylates, and verapamil.

Procedure and patient care

Before

- Discuss with the patient the need and reason for frequent venipunctures in diagnosing MI.
- Avoid giving the patient any IM injection.
- If possible, hold drugs that could interfere with test results for 12 hours before the test.

During

- Collect a venous sample of blood in a red-top tube. This is usually done daily for 3 days and then again in 1 week.
- Rotate the venipuncture site.
- Avoid hemolysis.
- Record the exact time and date when the blood test is performed. This aids in the interpretation of the temporal pattern of enzyme elevations.

After

- Apply pressure to the venipuncture site.

Abnormal findings

▲ Increased levels

Heart diseases
Myocardial infarction
Cardiac operations
Cardiac catheterization and
  angioplasty
Liver diseases
Hepatitis
Hepatic cirrhosis
Drug-induced liver injury
Hepatic metastasis
Hepatic necrosis (initial
  stages only)
Hepatic surgery
Infectious mononucleosis
  with hepatitis
Hepatic infiltrative process
  (e.g., tumor)
Skeletal muscle diseases
Skeletal muscle trauma
Recent noncardiac surgery
Multiple traumas
Severe, deep burns
Progressive muscular
  dystrophy
Recent convulsions
Heat stroke
Primary muscle diseases
  (e.g., myopathy, myositis)
Other diseases
Acute hemolytic anemia
Acute pancreatitis

▼ Decreased levels
Acute renal disease
Beriberi
Diabetic ketoacidosis
Pregnancy
Chronic renal dialysis

notes

barium enema (BE, Lower GI series)

Type of test X-ray with contrast dye

Normal findings

Normal filling, contour, patency, and positioning of barium in the colon

Normal filling of the appendix and terminal ileum

Test explanation

The BE study consists of a series of x-ray films visualizing the colon. It is used to demonstrate the presence and location of polyps, tumors, and diverticula. Anatomic abnormalities (e.g., malrotation) also can be detected. Therapeutically BE may be used to reduce nonstrangulated ileocolic intussusception in children. Bleeding from diverticula can cease with barium enema.

BE is occasionally used to assess filling of the appendix. Although the colon is the main organ evaluated by a BE, reflux of barium into the terminal ileum also allows adequate visualization of the distal part of the small intestine. Diseases that affect the terminal ileum, especially Crohn's disease (regional enteritis), can be identified. Inflammatory bowel disease involving the colon can be detected with BE. Fistulas involving the colon can be demonstrated by BE.

In many instances, air is insufflated into the colon after the instillation of barium. This provides an air contrast to the barium. With air contrast, the colonic mucosa can be much more accurately visualized. This is called an *air-contrast barium enema.*

Contraindications

- Patients suspected of a perforation of the colon. In these patients diatrizoate (Gastrografin), a water-soluble contrast medium, is used.
- Patients who are unable to cooperate. This test requires the patient to hold the barium in the rectum and colon. This is especially difficult for elderly patients.
- Patients with megacolon. Barium may worsen the disease.

Potential complications

- Colonic perforation, especially when the colon is weakened by inflammation, tumor, or infection
- Barium fecal impaction

Interfering factors

- Barium within the abdomen from previous barium tests
- Significant residual stool within the colon. This precludes adequate visualization of the entire bowel wall. Stool may be confused for polyps.
- Spasm of the colon. Spasm can mimic the radiographic signs of a cancer. The use of IV glucagon minimizes spasm.

Procedure and patient care

Before

- Assist the patient with bowel preparation, which varies among institutions. In elderly patients this preparation can be exhaustive and even cause severe dehydration.
- Note that pediatric patients will have individualized bowel preparations.
- Note that special preparations will be ordered for patients with an ileostomy or colostomy.

During

- The test begins with placement of a balloon rectal catheter.
- The balloon on the catheter is inflated tightly against the anal sphincter to hold the barium within the colon.
- The patient is asked to roll in the lateral, supine, and prone positions.
- The barium is dripped into the rectum by gravity.
- The barium flow is monitored fluoroscopically.
- The colon is thoroughly examined as the barium flow progresses through the large colon and into the terminal ileum.
- The barium is drained out.
- If an air-contrast BE has been ordered, air is insufflated into the large bowel.
- The patient is asked to expel the barium, and a post-evacuation x-ray film is taken.
- Note that this test is usually performed in the radiology department by a radiologist in approximately 45 minutes.
- Inform the patient that abdominal bloating and rectal pressure will occur during instillation of barium.

After

- Ensure that the patient defecates as much barium as possible.
- Inform the patient that bowel movements will be white.

When all the barium has been expelled, the stool will return to normal color.

- Suggest the use of soothing ointments on the anal area to minimize any anorectal pain that may result from the aggressive test preparation.
- Encourage ingestion of fluids to avoid dehydration caused by the cathartics.
- Note that laxatives may be ordered to facilitate evacuation of barium.

Abnormal findings

Malignant tumor
Polyps
Diverticula
Inflammatory bowel diseases (e.g., ulcerative colitis, Crohn's disease)
Colonic stenosis secondary to ischemia, infection, or previous surgery
Perforated colon
Colonic fistula

Appendicitis
Extrinsic compression of the colon from extracolonic tumors (e.g., ovarian)
Extrinsic compression of the colon from an abscess
Malrotation of the gut
Colon volvulus
Intussusception
Hernia

notes

bilirubin, blood

Type of test Blood

Normal findings

Adult/elderly/child

Total bilirubin: 0.1-1 mg/dl or 5.1-17 μmol/L (SI units)

Indirect bilirubin: 0.2-0.8 mg/dl or 3.4-12.0 μmol/L (SI units)

Direct bilirubin: 0.1-0.3 mg/dl or 1.7-5.1 μmol/L (SI units)

Newborn total bilirubin: 1-12 mg/dl or 17.1-20.5 μmol/L (SI units)

Test explanation

Hemoglobin is released from red blood cells (RBCs) and broken down to heme and globin molecules. Heme is then catabolized to form biliverdin, which is transformed to bilirubin. This form of bilirubin is called *unconjugated (indirect) bilirubin*. In the liver, indirect bilirubin is conjugated with a glucuronide, resulting in *conjugated (direct) bilirubin*. The conjugated bilirubin is then excreted from the liver cells and into the intrahepatic canaliculi, which eventually lead to the hepatic ducts, the common bile duct, and the bowel.

Once jaundice is recognized either clinically or chemically (bilirubin exceeds 2.5 mg/dl), it is important (for therapy) to differentiate whether it is predominantly caused by unconjugated or conjugated bilirubin. This in turn will help differentiate the etiology of the defect. In general, jaundice caused by hepatocellular dysfunction (e.g., hepatitis) results in elevated levels of unconjugated bilirubin. Jaundice resulting from extrahepatic obstruction of the bile ducts (e.g., gallstones or tumor blocking the bile ducts) results in elevated conjugated bilirubin levels; this type of jaundice usually can be resolved surgically or endoscopically.

The total serum bilirubin level is the sum of the conjugated (direct) and unconjugated (indirect) bilirubin. These are separated out when "fractionation or differentiation" of the total bilirubin to its direct and indirect parts is requested. Normally the unconjugated bilirubin makes up 70% to 85% of the total bilirubin. In patients with jaundice, when more than 50% of the bilirubin is conjugated, it is considered a conjugated hyperbilirubinemia from gallstones, tumor, inflammation, scarring, or obstruction of the extrahepatic ducts. Unconjugated hyperbilirubinemia exists when less than 15% to 20% of the total bilirubin is conjugated. Diseases that typically cause this form of jaundice include accelerated erythrocyte (RBC) hemolysis, hepatitis, or drugs.

Interfering factors

- Blood hemolysis and lipemia can produce erroneous results.
- Drugs that may cause *increased* levels of total bilirubin include allopurinol, antibiotics, antimalarials, chlorpropamide (Diabinese), monoamine oxidase inhibitors, phenothiazines, rifampin, and vitamin A.

Procedure and patient care

Before

- Note that fasting requirements vary among different laboratories. Some require keeping the patient NPO after midnight the day of the test except for water.

During

- Collect 5 to 7 ml of venous blood in a red-top tube.
- Use a heel puncture for blood collection in infants.
- Prevent hemolysis of blood during phlebotomy.
- Protect the blood sample from bright light. Prolonged exposure (over 1 hour) to sunlight or artificial light can reduce bilirubin content.

After

- Apply pressure to the venipuncture site. Patients who are jaundiced can have prolonged clotting times.

Abnormal findings

▲ **Increased levels of conjugated (direct) bilirubin**

Gallstones

Extrahepatic duct obstruction (tumor, inflammation, gallstone, scarring, or surgical trauma)

Extensive liver metastasis

Cholestasis from drugs

Dubin-Johnson syndrome

Rotor's syndrome

▲ **Increased levels of unconjugated (indirect) bilirubin**

Erythroblastosis fetalis

Hemolytic jaundice

Large-volume blood transfusion

Resolution of a large hematoma

Hepatitis

Sepsis

Neonatal hyperbilirubinemia

Hemolytic anemia

Crigler-Najjar syndrome

Gilbert syndrome

Pernicious anemia

Cirrhosis

Transfusion reaction

Sickle cell anemia

notes

bleeding time (Ivy bleeding time)

Type of test Blood

Normal findings 1-9 minutes (Ivy method) (results vary among laboratories)

Possible critical values >12 minutes

Test explanation

The bleeding time test is used to evaluate the vascular and platelet factors associated with hemostasis. It is frequently performed on preoperative patients to ensure adequate hemostasis. When vascular injury occurs, the first hemostatic response is a spastic contraction of the lacerated microvessels. Next, platelets adhere to the wall of the vessel at the area of laceration in an attempt to plug the hole. Failure of either process results in a prolonged bleeding time. If platelets are present in inadequate quantities (usually less than $50,000/mm^3$), if the platelet function is inadequate (as in patients with uremia or with recent ingestion of aspirin), or if vessel constriction is inadequate (such as exists in the elderly or with increased capillary fragility), the bleeding time is prolonged.

For this study a small, standard superficial incision is made in the forearm, and the time required for the bleeding to stop is recorded. This is called the *bleeding time*. Normal values vary according to the method used; the method most often used today is the Ivy bleeding time test.

Potential complications

- Skin infection
- Excessive bleeding from test site

Interfering factors

- Aggressively wiping the site of laceration can prolong the test results.
- Extremes in body temperatures can alter results. High temperatures can prolong results, low body temperatures can fictitiously shorten results.
- ✔ Drugs that may cause *increased* bleeding times include anticoagulants, dextran, salicylates, allopurinol, nonsteroidal antiinflammatory drugs, and urokinase.

Procedure and patient care

Before

- Obtain a drug history to detect if the patient has recently had aspirin, anticoagulants, or any other medications that may affect test results.
- Inform the patient that minor discomfort may occur with this test because of the skin laceration.

During

- A blood pressure cuff is applied on the arm above the elbow, inflated to 40 mm Hg, and maintained at this pressure during the study.
- A small laceration is then made 1-mm deep into the skin, and the time is recorded.
- Bleeding ensues, and the blood is wiped clean at 30-second intervals.
- When no new bleeding occurs, the time is again noted.
- The interval from the beginning to the end of bleeding is calculated. This is the bleeding time.
- If bleeding persists more than 10 minutes, the test is stopped, and a pressure dressing is applied.
- Note that this test is usually performed by a laboratory technician in less than 10 minutes.

After

- Abnormal results should be repeated.

Abnormal findings

▲   **Prolonged times or increased values**

Bone marrow failure	Henoch-Schönlein syndrome
Primary or metastatic tumor infiltration of bone marrow	Severe liver disease
	Clotting factor deficiency
	Capillary fragility
Disseminated intravascular coagulation	Leukemia
	Uremia
Thrombocytopenia	Bernard-Soulier syndrome
Hypersplenism	Connective tissue disorder
von Willebrand's disease	Hereditary telangiectasia
Collagen vascular disease	Glanzmann's thrombasthenia
Cushing syndrome	

blood typing

B

Type of test Blood

Normal findings Compatibility

Test explanation

With blood typing, ABO and Rh antigens can be detected in the blood of prospective blood donors and potential blood recipients. This test is also used to determine the blood type of expectant mothers and newborns.

ABO system

Human blood is grouped according to the presence or absence of A or B antigens. The surface membrane of group A red blood cells (RBCs) contains A antigens; group B RBCs contain B antigens on their surface; group AB RBCs have both A and B antigens; and group O RBCs have neither A nor B antigens. A person's serum does not contain antibodies to match the surface antigen on their RBCs. Blood transfusions are actually transplantations of tissue (blood) from one person to another. It is important that the recipient not have antibodies to the donor's RBCs. If this were to occur, there could be a hypersensitivity reaction, which can vary from mild fever to anaphylaxis with severe intravascular hemolysis. If donor ABO antibodies are present against the recipient antigens, usually only minimal reactions occur.

Rh factors

The presence or absence of Rh antigens on the RBCs surface determines the classification of Rh positive or Rh negative. The major Rh factor is Rh_o (D). There are several minor Rh factors. If Rh_o (D) is absent, the minor Rh antigens are tested. If negative, the patient is considered "Rh negative" (Rh_).

Procedure and patient care

Before
- Tell the patient that no fasting is required.

During
- Collect approximately 7 to 14 ml of venous blood in a red-top tube. (This may vary among laboratories.)
- Avoid hemolysis

- Appropriately label the blood tube before sending it to the laboratory.

After

- Assess the venipuncture site for bleeding.

Abnormal findings

See Test Explanation.

notes

bone densitometry (Bone mineral content [BMC], Bone absorptiometry, Bone mineral density [BMD])

Type of test X-ray

Normal findings

Normal: <1 standard deviation below normal (>−1)
Osteopenia: 1-2.5 standard deviations below normal (−1 to −2.5)
Osteoporosis: >2.5 standard deviations below normal (<−2.5)

Test explanation

Bone densitometry to determine bone mineral content and density is used to diagnose osteoporosis as early as possible. *Osteoporosis/osteopenia* are terms used for bone that becomes weakened and fractures easily. There are other diseases in patients that are associated with osteoporosis such as malnourishment or osteopenic endocrinopathies (e.g., hyperparathyroidism). Bone densitometry can provide early and accurate measurement of bone strength based on bone density.

Several groups of bones are routinely evaluated because they accurately represent the entire skeleton. The lumbar spine is the best representative of cancellous bone. The radius is the most easily studied cortical bone. The proximal hip (neck of the femur) is the best representative of mixed (cancellous and cortical) bone.

Dual-energy densitometry (absorptiometry) is most commonly used. There are two different types of dual photon energy and therefore two different methods of performing dual-energy densitometry. *Dual-photon absorptiometry (DPA)* and *dual-energy x-ray absorptiometry (DEXA)* are most commonly used. Because DPA and DEXA use two photons, more energy is produced so that bones (spine and hip [femoral neck]) surrounded by a lot of soft tissue can be more easily penetrated. The source of the photon is placed on one side of the bone to be studied. The gamma detector is placed on the other side. Increased bone density is associated with increased bone photon absorption and, therefore, less photon recognition at the site of the gamma detector.

The diagnosis of osteoporosis can be made when vertebral bone density is more than 10% below that expected according to a chart based on sex, age, height, weight, and race. Usually bone density is reported in terms of standard deviation (SD) removed from mean values. T scores compare the patient's results to a group of young healthy adults. Z scores compare the patient's results to a group of age-matched controls. The World Health Organization has defined osteopenia as a bone density value of >1 SD below peak bone mass levels recorded in young women and osteoporosis as a value of >2.5 SD below that same measurement scale. Positive T scores indicate bone stronger than normal. Negative T scores indicate bone weaker than normal.

This test is also used to monitor patients who are undergoing treatment for osteoporosis.

Interfering factors

- Barium may falsely increase the density of the lumbar spine. Bone density measurements should not be performed for about 10 days after barium studies.
- Calcified abdominal aortic aneurysm may falsely increase bone density of the spine.
- Internal fixation devices of the hip or radius will falsely increase bone density of those bones.
- Overlying metal jewelry or other objects may falsely increase bone density of the bones.
- Previous fractures of the bone to be studied can falsely increase bone density of the bone.
- Metallic clips placed in the plane of the vertebra of patients who have had previous abdominal surgery can falsely increase bone density of the bone.
- Prior bone scans can falsely decrease bone density because the photons generated from the bone (as a result of the previously administered bone scan radionuclide) will be detected by the scintillator detector.

Procedure and patient care

Before

- Tell the patient that no fasting or sedation is required.
- The machine is usually calibrated by the x-ray or nuclear medicine technician before the patient's arrival.
- Ask the patient to remove all metallic objects (e.g., belt buckles, zippers, coins, keys) that might be in the scanning path.

During

- Note the following procedural steps:
  1. The patient lies on an imaging table with the legs supported and placed on a padded box to flatten the pelvis and lumbar spine.
  2. Under the table, a photon generator is slowly successively passed under the lumbar spine.
  3. A scintillator (gamma or x-ray) detector/camera is passed over the patient in a manner parallel to the generator. An image of the lumbar spine and hip bone is obtained by the scintillator camera and projected on a computer monitor.
  4. Next, the patient's foot is applied to a brace that internally rotates the nondominant hip, and the procedure is repeated over the hip. The similar procedure is performed for radius evaluation.
  5. When the radius is examined, the nondominant arm is preferred, unless there is a history of fracture to that bone.
- Note that the data are interpreted by a radiologist or a physician trained in nuclear medicine.
- Note that bone density studies take about 30 to 45 minutes to perform and are free of any discomfort. Only minimal radiation is used for this procedure.

After

- On the computer screen, a small window of the lumbar spine, femoral neck, or distal radius is drawn. The computer calculates the amount of photons not absorbed by the bone. This is called the bone mineral content (BMC).

Abnormal findings

Osteopenia
Osteoporosis

notes

bone marrow biopsy (Bone marrow examination, Bone marrow aspiration)

Type of test Microscopic examination of tissue

Normal findings

Cell type	Range (%)
Myeloblasts	<5
Promyelocytes	1-8
Myelocytes	
Neutrophilic	5-15
Eosinophilic	0.5-3
Basophilic	<1
Metamyelocytes	
Neutrophilic	15-25
Eosinophilic	<1
Basophilic	<1
Mature myelocytes	
Neutrophilic	10-30
Eosinophilic	<5
Basophilic	<5
Mononuclear	
Monocytes	<5
Lymphocytes	3-20
Plasma cells	<1
Megakaryocytes	<5
M/E ratio	<4
Normoblasts	25-50

Normal iron content is demonstrated by staining with Prussian blue

Test explanation

Bone marrow examination is an important part of the evaluation of patients with hematologic diseases. Indications for bone marrow examination include the following:

1. To confirm the diagnosis of megaloblastic anemias
2. To diagnose leukemia or myeloma
3. To determine if the marrow is the cause of reduced blood cells in the peripheral bloodstream

4. To document deficient iron stores
5. To document bone marrow infiltrative diseases (neoplasm or fibrosis)
6. To identify a tumor, as in staging lymphomas

The bone marrow is located in the central fatty core of cancellous bone (sternum, rib, and pelvis) and the long bones (femur, tibia, and humerus).

By examination of a bone marrow specimen, the hematologist can fully evaluate hematopoiesis. Examination of the bone marrow reveals the number, size, and shape of the red and white blood cells (RBCs, WBCs) and megakaryocytes (platelet precursors) as these cells evolve through their various stages of development in the bone marrow. Microscopic examination includes estimation of cellularity, determination of the presence of fibrotic tissue or neoplasms (both primary and metastatic), and estimation of iron storage.

Leukemias or leukemoid drug reactions are suspected when increased numbers of leukocyte precursors are present. Decreased numbers of marrow leukocyte precursors occur in patients with myelofibrosis, metastatic neoplasia, or agranulocytosis; in elderly patients; and following radiation therapy or chemotherapy.

Increased numbers of marrow RBC precursors occur with polycythemia vera or as physiologic compensation to hypoxemia or hemorrhagic or hemolytic anemias. Decreased numbers of marrow RBC precursors occur with erythroid hypoplasia following chemotherapy, radiation therapy, administration of other toxic drugs, iron deficiency, or marrow replacement by fibrotic tissue or neoplasms.

Increased numbers of platelet precursors (megakaryocytes) are seen in the marrow of patients who are compensating after an episode of acute hemorrhage. They are also seen in some forms of chronic myeloid leukemia. Decreased numbers of megakaryocytes occur in patients who have had radiation therapy, chemotherapy, or other drug therapy and in patients with neoplastic or fibrotic marrow infiltrative diseases. Patients with aplastic anemia also have decreased numbers of megakaryocytes.

Increased numbers of lymphocyte precursors occur in chronic, viral, or mycoplasma infections (e.g., mononucleosis), lymphocytic leukemia, and lymphoma. Plasma cells (plasmocytes) are increased in number in patients with multiple myelomas, Hodgkin's disease, hypersensitivity states, rheumatic fever, and other chronic inflammatory diseases.

Estimation of cellularity also can be expressed as a ratio of myeloid (WBC) to erythroid (RBC) cells (M/E ratio). The normal M/E ratio is approximately 3:1. The M/E ratio is greater than normal in those diseases mentioned previously in which increased leukocyte precursors are present or erythroid precursors are decreased. The M/E ratio is below normal when either leukocyte precursors are decreased or erythroid precursors are increased.

Contraindications

- Patients with acute coagulation disorders because of the risk of excessive bleeding
- Patients who cannot cooperate and remain still during the procedure

Potential complications

- Hemorrhage, especially if the patient has a coagulopathy
- Infection, especially if the patient is leukopenic
- Sternal fracture as a result of too aggressive application of pressure to the sternum at the time of biopsy
- Inadvertent puncture of the heart or great vessels when the test is performed on the sternum

Procedure and patient care

Before

- Encourage the patient to verbalize fears because many patients are anxious concerning this study.
- Assess the coagulation studies. Report any evidence of coagulopathy to the physician.

During

- Note the following procedural steps for *bone marrow aspiration,* which is performed on the sternum, iliac crest, anterior or posterior iliac spines, and proximal tibia (in children):
  1. A preferred site is the posterior iliac crest, with the patient placed prone or on the side.
  2. The overlying skin and soft tissue, along with the periosteum, is infiltrated with lidocaine.
  3. A large-bore needle containing a stylus is slowly advanced through the soft tissue and into the outer table of the bone.
  4. One half to 2 ml of bone marrow is aspirated, smeared on slides, and allowed to dry.
- Note the following procedural steps for *bone marrow biopsy:*
  1. A core biopsy instrument is "screwed" into the bone.

2. The biopsy specimen is obtained and sent to the pathology laboratory for analysis.

- Note that aspiration is performed by a trained nurse or physician. Bone marrow biopsy is usually performed by a physician. The duration of these studies is approximately 20 minutes.
- Tell the patient that he or she probably will feel pain during lidocaine infiltration and pressure when the syringe plunger is withdrawn for aspiration.

After

- Apply pressure to the puncture site to arrest minimal bleeding. Apply an adhesive bandage.
- Normally place the patient on bed rest for 30 to 60 minutes after the test.
- Note that some patients complain of tenderness at the puncture site for several days after this study. Mild analgesics may be ordered.

Abnormal findings

Neoplasm
Viral infection
Bacterial infection
Fungal infection
Myelofibrosis
Agranulocytosis
Polycythemia vera
Multiple myelomas
Hodgkin's disease
Hypersensitivity states

Acute hemorrhagic marrow hyper-
   plasia
Anemia
Lymphoma
Chronic inflammatory disease
Leukemia
Rheumatic fever
AIDS

notes

bone scan

Type of test Nuclear scan

Normal findings No evidence of abnormality

Test explanation

The bone scan permits examination of the skeleton by a scanning camera after IV injection of a radionuclide material. Usually technetium (Tc)-99m is the radionuclide used.

The degree of radionuclide uptake is related to the metabolism of the bone. Normally a uniform concentration should be seen throughout the bones of the body. An increased uptake of isotope is abnormal and may represent tumor, arthritis, fracture, degenerative bone and joint changes, osteomyelitis, bone necrosis, osteodystrophy, or Paget's disease.

The major reason a bone scan is performed is to detect metastatic cancer to the bone. All malignancies capable of metastasis may reach the bone, especially those of the prostate, breast, lung, kidney, urinary bladder, and thyroid gland. Bone scans may be serially repeated to monitor tumor response to antineoplastic therapy.

Bone scans also provide valuable information in the evaluation of patients with trauma or unexplained pain. Bone scanning is much more sensitive than routine x-ray films in detecting small and difficult-to-find fractures, especially in the spine, ribs, face, and small bones of the extremities. Bone scans are used to determine the age of a fracture as well.

Although the bone scan is extremely sensitive, unfortunately it is not very specific. Fractures, infections, tumors, and arthritic changes all appear similar in this scan. Bone scans are helpful in identifying infection (osteomyelitis) when plain films fail to identify the classic findings of infection.

Contraindications

- Patients who are pregnant because of risk of fetal damage
- Patients who are lactating because of risk of contaminating the infant

Procedure and patient care

Before

- Assure patients they will not be exposed to large amounts of radioactivity because only tracer doses of the isotope are used.
- Tell the patient that no fasting or sedation is required.

During

- Note the following procedural steps:
  1. The patient receives an IV injection of an isotope, usually sodium pertechnetate (technetium-99m) in a peripheral vein.
  2. The patient is encouraged to drink several glasses of water between the time of radioisotope injection and the scanning. This facilitates renal clearance of the circulating tracer not picked up by the bone. The waiting period before scanning is approximately 1 to 3 hours.
  3. The patient is instructed to urinate.
  4. The patient is positioned in the supine position on the scanning table in the nuclear medicine department.
  5. A radionuclide detector is placed over the patient's body and records the radiation emitted by the skeleton.
  6. The patient is repositioned in the prone and lateral positions during the test.
- Note that this scan is performed by a nuclear medicine technician in 30 to 60 minutes. It is interpreted by a physician trained in nuclear medicine imaging.

After

- Because only tracer doses of radioisotope are used, remember that no precautions need to be taken to prevent radioactive exposure to other personnel or family present.
- Assure the patient that the radioactive substance is usually excreted from the body within 6 to 24 hours.
- Encourage the patient to drink fluids to aid in the excretion of the radioactive substance.

Abnormal findings

Primary or metastatic tumor of the bone
Fracture
Degenerative arthritis
Rheumatoid arthritis
Osteomyelitis
Bone necrosis
Renal osteodystrophy
Paget's disease
Osteomyelitis

BONE X-RAY

long bones x-ray
spine x-ray

Type of test X-ray

Normal findings No evidence of malposition, fracture, tumor, infection, or congenital abnormalities

Test explanation

X-ray films of the bones are usually taken when the patient has complaints about a particular body area. Fractures or tumors are readily detected by x-ray studies. In patients who have a severe or chronic infection overlying a bone, an x-ray film may detect the infection involving that bone (osteomyelitis). X-ray studies of the long bones can also detect joint destruction and bone spurring as a result of persistent arthritis. Growth patterns can be followed by serial x-ray studies of a long bone, usually in the wrists and hands. Healing of a fracture can also be documented and followed. X-ray films of the joints reveal as well the presence of joint effusions and soft tissue swelling. Calcifications in the soft tissue indicate chronic inflammatory changes of the nearby bursa or tendons. Soft tissue swelling can also be seen on bone x-rays.

Spinal films are often done to assess back or neck pain, degenerative arthritic changes, traumatic fractures, tumor metastasis, spondylosis (stress fracture of the vertebrae), and spondylolisthesis (slipping of one vertebral disk on the other). Cervical spine x-ray studies are routinely performed in cases of multiple trauma to ensure there is no fracture before the patient is moved or the neck is manipulated. Spinal x-rays are very helpful in evaluating children and adults for spinal alignment abnormalities (e.g., kyphosis, scoliosis).

Interfering factors

- Jewelry or clothing can obstruct radiographic visualization of part of the bone to be evaluated.
- Prior barium studies can diminish the full radiographic visualization of some of the bones surrounding the abdomen (e.g., spine, and pelvis).

Procedure and patient care

Before

- Explain the procedure to the patient.
- Handle carefully any injured areas of the patient's body.
- Instruct the patient that he or she will need to keep the extremity still while the x-ray film is being taken. This can sometimes be difficult, especially when the patient has severe pain associated with a recent injury.
- Shield the patient's testes, ovaries, or pregnant abdomen to avoid exposure from scattered radiation.
- Immobilize the patient if a spinal fracture is suspected. Apply a neck brace if a cervical spine fracture is suspected.

During

- Note that the patient is placed on an x-ray table. Anterior, posterior, lateral, and oblique x-ray films are taken of the desired area.

After

- Note that positioning and patient activity depend on test results.

Abnormal findings

Fractures
Congenital bone disorders
  (e.g., achondroplasia,
  dysplasia, dysostosis)
Tumors (osteogenic sarcoma,
  Paget's disease, myeloma,
  or metastases)
Infection/osteomyelitis
Osteoporosis/osteopenia

Joint destruction (arthritis)
Bone spurring
Abnormal growth pattern
Joint effusion
Spondylosis
Spondylolisthesis
Foreign bodies

notes

breast sonogram (Ultrasound mammography)

Type of test Ultrasound

Normal findings No evidence of cyst or tumor

Test explanation

This ultrasound examination of the breast is most commonly used to determine if a mammographic abnormality or a palpable lump is a cyst (fluid-filled) or solid tumor (benign or malignant). Ultrasound of the breast is also useful in the examination of symptomatic women for whom the radiation of mammography is potentially harmful.

Diagnostic accuracy is improved when breast ultrasound is combined with x-ray mammography (see p. 199). Ultrasound can be used to locate a nonpalpable breast abnormality for biopsy or aspiration.

Procedure and patient care

Before

- Assure the patient that no discomfort is associated with this study.
- Inform the patient that no fasting or sedation is required before the tests.

During

- Note the following procedural steps:
  1. The patient lies in the prone position on the examining table, which contains a tank that holds heated and chlorinated water.
  2. One breast at a time is immersed in the water.
  3. The transducer that produces the ultrasound waves and detects their echoes is positioned at the bottom of the water tank.
  4. Alternatively the patient is placed in the supine position, and the transducer is directly applied to the breast using contact gel to improve sound transmission.
- Note that this test is performed by an ultrasound technician in approximately 15 minutes.

After

- After the test is completed, the breasts are dried, and the conductive paste is removed.

Abnormal findings

Cyst	Fibroadenoma
Hematoma	Fibrocystic disease
Cancer	Abscess

notes

bronchoscopy

Type of test Endoscopy

Normal findings Normal larynx, trachea, bronchi, and alveoli

Test explanation

Bronchoscopy permits endoscopic visualization of the larynx, trachea, and bronchi by either a flexible fiberoptic bronchoscope or a rigid bronchoscope. There are many diagnostic and therapeutic uses for bronchoscopy. *Diagnostic* uses of bronchoscopy include:

1. Direct visualization of the tracheobronchial tree for abnormalities (e.g., tumors, inflammation, strictures)
2. Biopsy of tissue from observed lesions
3. Aspiration of "deep" sputum for culture and sensitivity and for cytology determinations
4. Direct visualization of the larynx for identification of vocal cord paralysis, if present

Therapeutic uses of bronchoscopy include:

1. Aspiration of retained secretions in patients with airway obstruction or postoperative atelectasis
2. Control of bleeding within the bronchus
3. Removal of foreign bodies that have been aspirated
4. Brachytherapy, which is endobronchial radiation therapy using an iridium wire placed via the bronchoscope
5. Palliative laser obliteration of bronchial neoplastic obstruction

Contraindications

- Patients with hypoxemia and severe shortness of breath who cannot tolerate interruption of high-flow oxygen (however, bronchoscopy can be performed through a special oxygen mask or an endotracheal tube so that the patient can receive oxygen if required)
- Patients with severe tracheal stenosis that may make it difficult to pass a scope

Potential complications

- Fever
- Hypoxemia
- Laryngospasm

- Bronchospasm
- Pneumothorax
- Aspiration
- Hemorrhage (after biopsy)

Procedure and patient care

Before

- Obtain informed consent for this procedure.
- Keep the patient NPO for 4 to 8 hours before the test to reduce the risk of aspiration.
- Instruct the patient to perform good mouth care to minimize the risk of introducing bacteria into the lungs during the procedure.
- Remove and safely store the patient's dentures, glasses, or contact lenses before administering the preprocedural medications.
- Reassure the patient that he or she will be able to breathe during this procedure.
- Instruct the patient not to swallow the local anesthetic sprayed into the throat. Provide a basin for expectoration of the lidocaine.

During

- Note the following procedural steps for *fiberoptic bronchoscopy:*
  1. This test is performed by a pulmonary specialist or a surgeon at the bedside or in an appropriately equipped room.
  2. The patient's nasopharynx and oropharynx are anesthetized topically with lidocaine spray before the insertion of the bronchoscope.
  3. The patient is placed in the sitting or supine position, and the tube is inserted through the nose or mouth and into the pharynx.
  4. After the bronchoscope passes into the larynx and through the glottis, more lidocaine is sprayed into the trachea to prevent the cough reflex.
  5. The scope is passed farther, well into the trachea, bronchi, and first- and second-generation bronchioles, for systematic examination of the bronchial tree.
  6. Biopsy specimens and washings are taken if pathology is suspected.

7. If bronchoscopy is performed for pulmonary toilet (removal of mucus), each bronchus is aspirated until clear.

- Note that this procedure is performed by a physician in approximately 30 to 45 minutes.

After

- Instruct the patient not to eat or drink anything until the tracheobronchial anesthesia has worn off and the gag reflex has returned, usually in approximately 2 hours.
- Observe the patient's sputum for hemorrhage if biopsy specimens were removed. A small amount of blood streaking may be expected and is normal for several hours.
- Observe the patient closely for evidence of impaired respiration or laryngospasm. The vocal cords may go into spasms after intubation.
- Inform the patient that postbronchoscopy fever often develops within the first 24 hours.
- If a tumor is suspected, collect a postbronchoscopy sputum sample for a cytology determination.
- Inform the patient that warm saline gargles and lozenges may be helpful if a sore throat develops.

Abnormal findings

Inflammation	Hemorrhage
Strictures	Foreign body
Tuberculosis	Abscess
Cancer	Infection

notes

calcium (Total/ionized calcium, Ca, Serum calcium)

Type of test Blood

Normal findings

Age	mg/dl	mmol/L
Total calcium		
<10 days	7.6-10.4	1.9-2.6
Umbilical	9-11.5	2.25-2.88
10 days-2 years	9-10.6	2.3-2.65
Child	8.8-10.8	2.2-2.7
Adult*	9-10.5	2.25-2.75
Ionized calcium		
Newborn	4.20-5.58	1.05-1.37
2 mos-18 yrs	4.80-5.52	1.20-1.38
Adult	4.5-5.6	1.05-1.3

*In the elderly, values tend to decrease.

Possible critical values

<6 mg/dl (may lead to tetany)
>14 mg/dl (may lead to coma)

Test explanation

The serum calcium test is used to evaluate parathyroid function and calcium metabolism by directly measuring the total amount of calcium in the blood. Determination of serum calcium is used to monitor patients with renal failure, renal transplantation, hyperparathyroidism, and various malignancies. It is also used to monitor calcium levels during and after large-volume blood transfusions.

About one half of the total calcium exists in the blood in its free (ionized) form, and about one half exists in its protein-bound form (mostly with albumin). The serum calcium level is a measure of both. As a result, when the serum albumin level is low (as in malnourished patients), the serum calcium level will also be low, and vice versa. As a rule of thumb, the total serum calcium level decreases by approximately 0.8 mg for every 1-g decrease in the serum albumin level. Serum albumin should be measured with serum calcium. An advantage of measuring only the ionized form is that it is unaffected by changes in serum albumin levels.

When the serum calcium level is elevated on at least three separate determinations, the patient is said to have hypercalcemia. The most common cause of hypercalcemia is hyperparathyroidism. Malignancy is the second most common cause of hypercalcemia. Cancer (lung, breast, renal cell) can produce a parathyroid hormone–like substance that drives the serum calcium up (ectopic PTH). Excess vitamin D ingestion can also increase serum calcium by increasing renal and gastrointestinal absorption. Granulomatous infections such as sarcoidosis or tuberculosis are also associated with hypercalcemia.

Hypocalcemia occurs in patients with hypoalbuminemia. Large blood transfusions are associated with low serum calcium levels because the citrate additives used in banked blood for anticoagulation bind the free calcium in the recipient's bloodstream. Intestinal malabsorption, renal failure, rhabdomyolysis, alkalosis, and acute pancreatitis (caused by saponification of fat) are also known to be associated with low serum calcium levels. Hypomagnesemia can be associated with refractory hypocalcemia.

Interfering factors

- Vitamin D intoxication may cause increased serum calcium levels.
- Serum pH can affect calcium values. A decrease in pH causes increased calcium levels.
- Prolonged tourniquet time will lower pH and factitiously increase calcium levels.
- Drugs that may cause *increased* serum levels include calcium salts, lithium, thiazide diuretics, parathyroid hormone (PTH), thyroid hormone, alkaline antacids, and vitamin D.
- Drugs that may cause *decreased* serum levels include acetazolamide, anticonvulsants, aspirin, calcitonin, corticosteroids, heparin, laxatives, loop diuretics, magnesium salts, diuretics, and albuterol.

Procedure and patient care

Before

- Tell the patient that no fasting is required; however, the serum calcium may be part of a multichemical analysis in which fasting is required for the other studies.

During
- Collect approximately 7 ml of venous blood in a red-top tube. Avoid prolonged tourniquet use.

After
- Apply pressure to the venipuncture site.

Abnormal findings

▲ **Increased levels (hypercalcemia)**
Hyperparathyroidism
Nonparathyroid PTH-producing tumor (e.g., lung or renal carcinoma)
Metastatic tumor to the bone
Paget's disease of the bone
Prolonged immobilization
Milk-alkali syndrome
Vitamin D intoxication
Lymphoma
Granulomatous infections (e.g., sarcoidosis and tuberculosis)
Addison's disease
Acromegaly
Hyperthyroidism

▼ **Decreased values (hypocalcemia)**
Hypoparathyroidism
Renal failure
Hyperphosphatemia secondary to renal failure
Rickets
Vitamin D deficiency
Osteomalacia
Malabsorption
Pancreatitis
Fat embolism
Alkalosis

notes

carbon dioxide content (CO_2 content, CO_2 combining power)

Type of test Blood

Normal findings

Adult/elderly: 23-30 mEq/L or 23-30 mmol/L (SI units)
Child: 20-28 mEq/L
Infant: 20-28 mEq/L
Newborn: 13-22 mEq/L

Possible critical values <6 mEq/L

Test explanation

The CO_2 content is a measure of CO_2 in the blood. In the peripheral venous blood, this is used to assist in evaluating the pH status of the patient and to assist in evaluation of electrolytes. The serum CO_2 test is usually included with other assessments of electrolytes. It is usually done with a multiphasic testing machine, which also measures sodium, potassium, chloride, BUN, and creatinine. It is important not to get this test confused with P_{CO_2}. This CO_2 content measures the H_2CO_3, dissolved CO_2, and bicarbonate ion (HCO_3^-) that exists in the serum. Because the amounts of H_2CO_3 and dissolved CO_2 in the blood are so small, CO_2 content is an indirect measure of HCO_3^- anion. HCO_3^- anion is second in importance to the chloride ion in electrical neutrality (negative charge) of extracellular and intracellular fluid; its major role is in acid-base balance. Increases occur with alkalosis, and decreases occur with acidosis.

Interfering factors

- Underfilling the tube with blood allows CO_2 to escape from the serum specimen and may significantly reduce HCO_3^- values.
- Drugs that may cause *increased* serum CO_2 and HCO_3^- levels include aldosterone, barbiturates, bicarbonates, loop diuretics, and steroids.
- Drugs that may cause *decreased* levels include thiazide diuretics and triamterene.

Procedure and patient care

Before
- Tell the patient that no fasting is required.

During
- Collect approximately 7 to 10 ml of venous blood in a red- or green-top tube.

After
- Apply pressure to the venipuncture site.

Abnormal findings

▲ **Increased levels**
Severe diarrhea
Starvation
Severe vomiting
Aldosteronism
Emphysema
Metabolic alkalosis
Gastric suction

▼ **Decreased levels**
Renal failure
Salicylate toxicity
Diabetic ketoacidosis
Metabolic acidosis
Shock
Starvation

notes

cardiac catheterization (Coronary angiography, Angiocardiography, Ventriculography)

Type of test   X-ray with contrast dye

Normal findings   Normal heart-muscle motion, normal coronary arteries, normal great vessels, and normal intracardiac pressures and volumes

Test explanation

Cardiac catheterization is used to visualize the heart chambers, arteries, and great vessels. It is used most often to evaluate patients with chest pain. Patients with a positive stress test are also studied to locate the region of coronary occlusion. This test is also used to determine the effects of valvular heart disease. Right heart catheterization is performed to calculate cardiac output. This is the most accurate method to determine cardiac output. Right heart catheterization is also used to identify pulmonary emboli.

For cardiac catheterization, a catheter is passed into the heart through a peripheral vein or artery, depending on whether catheterization of the right or left side of the heart is being performed. Pressures are recorded through the catheter, and radiographic dyes are injected. With the assistance of a computer, cardiac output and other measures of cardiac function can be determined. Cardiac catheterization is indicated for the following reasons:

1. To identify, locate, and quantitate the severity of atherosclerotic, occlusive coronary artery disease
2. To evaluate the severity of acquired and congenital cardiac valvular or septal defects
3. To determine the presence and degree of congenital cardiac abnormalities such as transposition of great vessels, patent ductus arteriosus, and anomalous venous return to the heart
4. To evaluate the success of previous cardiac surgery or balloon angioplasty
5. To evaluate cardiac muscle function
6. To identify and quantify ventricular aneurysms
7. To identify and locate acquired disease of the great vessels such as atherosclerotic occlusion or aneurysms within the aortic arch

8. To evaluate patients with acute myocardial infarction and facilitate infusion of thrombolytic agents into the occluded coronary arteries
9. To insert a catheter to monitor right-sided heart pressures such as pulmonary artery and pulmonary wedge pressures
10. To perform dilation of stenotic coronary arteries (angioplasty), place coronary artery stents, or perform laser atherectomy

Contraindications

- Patients who would refuse intervention if an amenable lesion were found
- Patients with an iodine dye allergy who have not received preventive medication for allergy
- Patients who are pregnant because of radiation exposure to the fetus
- Patients with renal disorders because iodinated contrast is nephrotoxic
- Patients with a bleeding propensity

Potential complications

- Cardiac arrhythmias (dysrhythmias)
- Perforation of the heart myocardium
- Catheter-induced embolic stroke (cerebrovascular accident) or myocardial infarction
- Complications associated with the catheter insertion site such as arterial thrombosis, embolism, infection, or pseudoaneurysm
- Possible hypoglycemia or acidosis in patients who are taking Glucophage and who receive iodine dye

Procedure and patient care

Before
- Obtain written permission from the fully informed patient.
- Allay the patient's fears and anxieties regarding this test. Although this test creates tremendous fear in a patient, it is performed often, and complications are rare.
- Instruct the patient to abstain from oral intake for at least 4 to 8 hours before the test.
- Prepare the catheter insertion site by shaving and scrubbing the skin.
- Mark the patient's peripheral pulses with a pen before cath-

eterization. This will facilitate postcatheterization assessment of the pulses at the affected and nonaffected extremities.

- Instruct the patient to void before going to the catheterization laboratory.
- Remove all valuables and dental prostheses before transporting the patient to the catheterization laboratory.
- Obtain IV access for delivery of IV fluids and cardiac drugs if necessary.

During

- Take the patient to the cardiac catheterization laboratory.
- Note the following procedural steps:
  1. The desired vessel is punctured with a needle.
  2. A wire is placed through the needle and into the catheter.
  3. The angiographic catheter is threaded on top of the wire.
  4. Once the catheter is in the desired location, the appropriate cardiac pressures and volumes are measured and contrast is injected.
  5. During the injection, x-ray films are rapidly made.
- Note that this test is usually performed by a cardiologist in approximately 1 hour.
- Tell the patient that during the injection he or she may experience a severe hot flush. This is uncomfortable but lasts only 10 to 15 seconds.

After

- Monitor the patient's vital signs.
- Apply pressure to the site of vascular access.
- Keep the patient on bed rest for 4 to 8 hours to allow for complete sealing of the arterial puncture.
- Keep the affected extremity extended and immobilized with sandbags to decrease bleeding.
- Assess the puncture site for signs of bleeding, hematoma, or absence of pulse.
- Assess the patient's pulses at both extremities. Compare with preprocedural baseline values.
- Encourage the patient to drink fluids to maintain adequate hydration. Dehydration may be caused by the diuretic action of the dye.

C

Abnormal findings

Anatomic variation of the cardiac chambers and great vessels
Coronary artery occlusive disease
Ventricular aneurysm
Ventricular mural thrombi
Intracardiac tumor
Aortic root arteriosclerotic or aneurysmal disease
Anomalies in pulmonary venous return
Acquired or congenital septal defects and valvular abnormalities
Pulmonary emboli
Pulmonary hypertension

notes

cardiac exercise stress testing (Stress testing; Exercise testing; Electrocardiograph [ECG] stress testing, Exercise testing; Nuclear stress testing, Echo stress testing)

Type of test Electrodiagnostic; nuclear

Normal findings Patient able to obtain and maintain maximal heart rate of 85% for predicted age and gender with no cardiac symptoms or ECG change. No cardiac muscle wall dysfunction present.

Test explanation

Stress testing is used in the following situations:

1. To evaluate chest pain in a patient suspected of having coronary disease (occasionally a person may have significant coronary stenosis that is not apparent during normal physical activity; if, however, the pain can be reproduced with exercise, one may infer that coronary occlusion is present)
2. To determine the limits of safe exercise during a cardiac rehabilitation program or to assist patients with cardiac disease in maintaining good physical fitness
3. To detect labile or exercise-related hypertension
4. To detect intermittent claudication in patients with suspected vascular occlusive disease in the extremities (in this situation, the patient may experience leg muscle cramping while performing the exercise)
5. To evaluate the effectiveness of treatment in patients who take antianginal or antiarrhythmic medications
6. To evaluate the effectiveness of cardiac intervention (such as bypass grafting or angioplasty)

Stress testing is a noninvasive study that provides information about the patient's cardiac function. In stress testing, the heart is stressed and then evaluated during the stress. Changes reflecting ischemia indicate coronary occlusive disease. By far the most commonly used method of stress is *exercise stress testing* (bike or treadmill). *Chemical stress testing* methods are becoming more commonly used because of their safety and increased accuracy. A third method, less commonly used, is *pacer stress testing*.

During *exercise stress testing*, ECG, heart rate, and blood pressure are monitored while the patient engages in some type of physical activity (stress). Two methods of stress testing include pedaling a stationary bike and walking on a treadmill. With the stationary bicycle, the pedaling tension is slowly increased to increase the heart rate. With the treadmill test, the speed and grade of incline are increased. The treadmill test is the most frequently used because it is the most easily standardized and reproducible. The various grades of exercise are determined by the cardiologist in attendance based on estimation of cardiac function capabilities.

The usual goal of exercise stress testing is to increase the heart rate to just below maximal levels or to the "target heart rate." Usually this target heart rate is 80% to 90% of the maximal heart rate. The test is usually discontinued if the patient reaches the target heart rate or develops any symptoms or ECG changes.

Exercise stress testing is based on the principle that occluded arteries will be unable to meet the heart's increased demand for blood during the testing. This may become obvious with symptoms (e.g., chest pain, fatigue, dyspnea, tachycardia, cardiac arrhythmias [dysrhythmias], fall in blood pressure) or ECG changes (e.g., ST-segment variance >1 mm, increasing premature ventricular contractions, or other rhythm disturbances). Besides the electrodiagnostic method of cardiac evaluation, the stressed heart can also be evaluated by nuclear scanning or echocardiography.

When exercise testing is not advisable or the patient is unable to exercise to a level adequate to stress the heart (patients with an orthopedic, arthritic, neurologic, or pulmonary limitation), *chemical stress testing* is recommended. Chemical stress testing is becoming increasingly used because of its accuracy and ease of performance. Although chemical stress testing is less physiologic than exercise testing, it is safer and more controllable. *Dipyridamole (Persantine)* is a coronary vasodilator. If one coronary artery is significantly occluded, the coronary blood flow is diverted to the opened vessels.

Adenosine works similarly to dipyridamole. *Dobutamine* is another chemical that can stress the heart. In chemical stress testing the stressed heart is evaluated by nuclear scanning or echocardiography.

Pacing is another method of stress testing. In patients with permanent pacemakers, the rate of capture can be increased to a rate that would be considered a cardiac stress.

The methods of evaluation of the heart are electrophysiologic (ECG) nuclear scanning and echocardiography.

Contraindications

- Patients with unstable angina
- Patients with severe aortic valvular heart disease
- Patients who have recently had a myocardial infarction (in this case, however, limited stress testing can be done)
- Patients with severe congestive heart failure

Potential complications

- Fatal cardiac arrhythmias
- Severe angina
- Myocardial infarction
- Fainting

Interfering factors

- Heavy meals before testing can divert blood to the gastrointestinal tract.
- Nicotine from smoking can cause coronary artery spasm.
- Medical problems such as left ventricular hypertrophy, hypertension, valvular heart disease (especially of the aortic valve), left bundle-branch block, severe anemia, hypoxemia, and chronic pulmonary disease can affect results.
- 🖋 Drugs that can affect test results include beta-blockers (e.g., propranolol [Inderal]), calcium channel blockers, digoxin, and nitroglycerine.

Procedure and patient care

Before

- Instruct the patient to abstain from eating, drinking, and smoking for 4 hours.
- Obtain informed consent.
- Instruct the patient to bring comfortable clothing and shoes in which to exercise. Slippers are not acceptable.
- Record the patient's vital signs for baseline values.
- Apply and secure appropriate ECG electrodes.

During

- Note that a physician usually is present during stress testing.
- After the patient begins to exercise, adjust the treadmill machine settings to apply increasing levels of stress at specific intervals.
- Note that during the test the ECG tracing and vital signs are monitored continuously.

- Terminate the test if the patient complains of chest pain, exhaustion, dyspnea, fatigue, or dizziness.
- Note that testing usually takes approximately 45 minutes.

After

- Place the patient in the supine position to rest after the test.
- Monitor the ECG tracing and record vital signs at post-stress intervals, until recordings and values return to pretest levels.

Abnormal findings

Coronary artery occlusive disease
Exercise-related hypertension
Intermittent claudication
Abnormal cardiac rhythms: stress-induced

notes

carotid duplex scanning

Type of test   Ultrasound

Normal findings   Carotid artery free of plaques and stenosis

Test explanation

Carotid duplex scanning is a noninvasive, ultrasound test used on the extracranial carotid artery to detect occlusive disease directly. It is recommended for patients with headaches and with neurologic symptoms such as transient ischemic attacks (TIA), hemiparesis, paresthesia, and acute speech or visual deficits.

The duplex scan can measure the amplitude and the wave form of the carotid arterial pulse. Furthermore, a two-dimensional image of the carotid artery can be produced. As a result, one can directly visualize possibly stenotic or occluded arteries and the arterial flow disruption.

Procedure and patient care

Before
- Tell the patient that no special preparation is required.
- Assure the patient that the study is painless.

During
- Place the patient in the supine position with the head supported to prevent lateral motion.
- Note the following procedural steps:
  1. A water-soluble gel is used to couple the sound from the transducer to the skin surface.
  2. Images of the carotid artery and pulse waveform are obtained.
- Note that this test is performed by an ultrasound technologist in the ultrasound or radiology department in approximately 15 to 30 minutes.
- Tell the patient that no discomfort is associated with this test.

After
- Remove the water-soluble gel from the patient.

Abnormal findings

Carotid artery occlusive disease

chest x-ray (CXR, Chest radiography)

Type of test X-ray

Normal findings Normal lungs and surrounding structures

Test explanation

The chest x-ray film is important in the complete evaluation of the pulmonary and cardiac systems. This procedure is often part of the general admission screening workup in adult patients. Much information can be provided by the chest x-ray film. One can identify or follow (by repeated chest x-ray films) the following:

1. Tumors of the lung (primary and metastatic), heart (myxoma), chest wall (soft tissue sarcomas), and bony thorax (osteogenic sarcoma)
2. Inflammation of the lung (pneumonia), pleura (pleuritis), and pericardium (pericarditis)
3. Fluid accumulation in the pleura (pleural effusion), pericardium (pericardial effusion), and lung (pulmonary edema)
4. Air accumulation in the lung (chronic obstructive pulmonary disease) and pleura (pneumothorax)
5. Fractures of the bones of the thorax or vertebrae
6. Diaphragmatic hernia
7. Heart size, which may vary depending on cardiac function
8. Calcification, which may indicate large-vessel deterioration or old lung granulomas
9. Location of centrally placed intravenous access devices

Most chest x-ray films are taken with the patient standing. The sitting or supine position also can be used, but x-ray films taken with the patient in the supine position will not demonstrate fluid levels. A *posteroanterior* (PA) view and a *lateral* view are taken. *Lordotic* views provide visualization of the apices of the lungs and are usually used for detection of tuberculosis. *Decubitus* films are taken with the patient in the recumbent lateral position to localize fluid.

Contraindications

- Patients who are pregnant

Interfering factors

- Conditions (e.g., severe pain) that prevent the patient from taking and holding a deep breath
- Scarring from previous lung surgery, which makes interpretation difficult
- Obesity, which requires more x-ray to penetrate the body to provide a readable picture

Procedure and patient care

Before

- Tell the patient that no fasting is required.
- Inform the patient to remove all metal objects (e.g., necklaces, pins) so that they do not block visualization of part of the chest.
- Instruct men to ensure that their testicles are covered and women to have their ovaries covered with a lead shield to prevent radiation-induced abnormalities.

During

- After the patient is correctly positioned, tell him or her to take a deep breath and hold it until the x-ray films are taken.
- Note that x-ray films are taken by a radiologic technologist in several minutes.

After

- Note that no special care is required following the procedure.

Abnormal findings

Lung

Lung tumor (primary or
   metastatic)
Pneumonia
Pulmonary edema
Pleural effusion
Chronic obstructive
   pulmonary disease
Pneumothorax
Atelectasis
Tuberculosis
Lung abscess
Congenital lung diseases
   (hypoplasia)
Pleuritis
Foreign bodies (chest, bron-
   chus, or esophagus)

Heart

Cardiac enlargement
Pericarditis
Pericardial effusion

Chest wall

Soft tissue sarcoma
Osteogenic sarcoma
Fracture (ribs or thoracic
   spine)
Thoracic spine scoliosis
Metastatic tumor to the bony
   thorax

Diaphragm

Diaphragmatic/hiatal
   hernia

Mediastinum

Aortic calcinosis
Enlarged lymph nodes
Dilated aorta
Thymoma
Lymphoma
Substernal thyroid
Widened mediastinum

notes

chloride, blood (Cl)

Type of test Blood

Normal findings

Adult/elderly: 90-110 mEq/L or 98-106 mmol/L (SI units)
Child: 90-110 mEq/L
Newborn: 96-106 mEq/L
Premature infant: 95-110 mEq/L

Possible critical values <80 or >115 mEq/L

Test explanation

This test is performed as a part of *multiphasic testing* in what is usually called "electrolytes." By itself, not much information is obtained. However, with interpretation of the other electrolytes, chloride can give an indication of acid-base balance and hydrational status.

Hypochloremia and hyperchloremia rarely occur alone and are usually part of parallel shifts in sodium or bicarbonate levels (see pp. 22 and 66). Signs and symptoms of hypochloremia include hyperexcitability of the nervous system and muscles, shallow breathing, hypotension, and tetany. Signs and symptoms of hyperchloremia include lethargy, weakness, and deep breathing.

Interfering factors

- Excessive infusions of saline can result in *increased* chloride levels.
- Drugs that may cause *increased* serum chloride levels include acetazolamide, chlorothiazide, and cortisone preparations.
- Drugs that may cause *decreased* levels include aldosterone, bicarbonates, corticosteroids, loop diuretics, thiazide diuretics, and triamterene.

Procedure and patient care

Before

- Tell the patient that no fasting is required.

During

- Collect 5 to 10 ml of venous blood in a red- or green-top tube.

After

- Apply pressure or a pressure dressing to the venipuncture site.

Abnormal findings

▲ **Increased levels (hyperchloremia)**
Dehydration
Renal tubular acidosis
Excessive infusion of normal saline
Cushing's syndrome
Eclampsia
Multiple myeloma
Kidney dysfunction
Metabolic acidosis
Hyperventilation
Anemia
Respiratory alkalosis
Hyperparathyroidism

▼ **Decreased levels (hypochloremia)**
Overhydration
Congestive heart failure
Syndrome of inappropriate secretion of antidiuretic hormone
Vomiting
Chronic gastric suction
Chronic respiratory acidosis
Salt-losing nephritis
Addison's disease
Burns
Metabolic alkalosis
Diuretic therapy
Hypokalemia
Aldosteronism
Respiratory acidosis

notes

cholesterol

Type of test Blood

Normal findings Vary with age and testing center
Adult/elderly: <200 mg/dl or <5.20 mmol/L (SI units)
Child: 120-200 mg/dl
Infant: 70-175 mg/dl
Newborn: 53-135 mg/dl

Test explanation

Cholesterol is the main lipid associated with arteriosclerotic vascular disease. However, cholesterol is required for the production of steroids, sex hormones, bile acids, and cellular membranes. Cholesterol is transported in the bloodstream by lipoproteins. Nearly 75% of the cholesterol is bound to low-density lipoproteins (LDLs) (see p. 178), and 25% is bound to high-density lipoproteins (HDLs) (see p. 178).

The purpose of cholesterol testing is to identify patients at risk for arteriosclerotic heart disease. Cholesterol testing is usually done as a part of *lipid profile* testing, which also evaluates lipoproteins (see p. 178) and triglycerides (see p. 266). There is considerable overlap in what are considered "normal" and "high-risk" levels. Because of these significant variabilities, elevated results should be corroborated by repeating the study. The two results should be averaged to obtain an accurate cholesterol for risk assessment.

Severe liver diseases and malnutrition are associated with low cholesterol levels. Familial hyperlipidemias and hyperlipoproteinemias are often associated with high cholesterol.

In 1984 the National Institutes of Health developed a consensus in regard to total cholesterol levels and risk of CHD (Table 1).

Interfering factors

- Pregnancy is usually associated with elevated cholesterol levels.
- Oophorectomy increases levels.
- Drugs that may cause *increased* levels include anabolic steroids, beta-adrenergic blocking agents, oral contraceptives, phenytoin (Dilantin), and thiazide diuretics.

TABLE 1 Total cholesterol as an indicator of risk of CHD (mg/100 ml [SI units: mmol/L])*

Age	Low risk	Moderate risk	High risk
2-19	<170 (4.4)	171-185	>185 (4.8)
20-29	<200 (5.5)	201-220	>220 (5.7)
30-39	<220 (5.7)	221-240	>240 (6.2)
>40	<240 (6.2)	241-260	>260 (6.8)

*When cholesterol testing is combined with lipoproteins, risk of CHD can be more accurately calculated.
From Pagana KD, Pagana TJ: *Mosby's manual of diagnostic and laboratory tests,* St Louis, 1998, Mosby.

☛ Drugs that may cause *decreased* levels include allopurinol, bile salt–binding agents, captopril, colchicine, colestipol, lovastatin (Mevacor), neomycin (oral), niacin, and other new cholesterol-lowering drugs.

Procedure and patient care

Before
- Instruct the patient to fast 12 to 14 hours after eating a low-fat diet before testing. Only water is permitted.
- Tell the patient that no alcohol should be taken 24 hours before the test.

During
- Collect 5 to 10 ml of blood in a red-top tube.
- Finger stick method is also often used in mass screening.

After
- Apply pressure to the venipuncture site.
- Instruct patients with high levels regarding a low-cholesterol diet, exercise, and appropriate body weight.

Abnormal findings

▲ **Increased levels**
Hypercholesterolemia
Hyperlipidemia
Hypothyroidism
Uncontrolled diabetes
  mellitus
Nephrotic syndrome
Pregnancy
High-cholesterol diet
Xanthomatosis
Hypertension
Myocardial infarction
Atherosclerosis
Biliary cirrhosis
Stress
Nephrosis

▼ **Decreased levels**
Malabsorption
Malnutrition
Hyperthyroidism
Cholesterol-lowering
  medication
Pernicious anemia
Hemolytic anemia
Sepsis
Stress
Liver disease
Acute myocardial infarc-
  tion

notes

colposcopy

Type of test Endoscopy

C

Normal findings Normal vagina and cervix

Test explanation

Colposcopy provides an in situ macroscopic examination of the vagina and cervix with a colposcope, which is a macroscope with a light source and a magnifying lens. With this procedure, tiny areas of dysplasia, carcinoma in situ, and invasive cancer that would be missed by the naked eye can be visualized, and biopsy specimens can be obtained. The study is performed on patients with abnormal vaginal epithelial patterns, cervical lesions, or suspicious Pap smear results.

One of the major advantages of this procedure is that of directing the biopsy to the area most likely to be truly representative of the lesion.

The need for up to 90% of cone biopsies is eliminated by an experienced colposcopist. Endocervical curettage may routinely accompany colposcopy to detect unknown lesions in the endocervical canal.

Contraindications

- Patients with heavy menstrual flow

Interfering factor

- Failure to cleanse the cervix of foreign materials (e.g., creams, medications) may impair visualization.

Procedure and patient care

Before

- Obtain informed consent if required by the institution.

During

- Note the following procedural steps:
  1. The patient is placed in the lithotomy position, and a vaginal speculum is used to expose the vagina and cervix.
  2. After the cervix is sampled for cytologic findings, it is cleansed with a 3% acetic acid solution to remove excess mucus and cellular debris. The acetic acid also accentuates the difference between normal and abnormal epithelial tissues.

3. The colposcope is focused on the cervix, which is then carefully examined.

4. Usually the entire lesion can be outlined and the most atypical areas selected for biopsy specimen removal.

- Note that colposcopy is performed by a physician in approximately 5 to 10 minutes.
- Tell the patient that some women complain of pressure pains from the vaginal speculum and that momentary discomfort may be felt if biopsy specimens are obtained.

After

- Inform the patient that she may have vaginal bleeding if biopsy specimens were taken. Suggest that she wear a sanitary pad.
- Instruct the patient to abstain from intercourse and not to insert anything (except a tampon) into the vagina until healing of a biopsy is confirmed.

Abnormal findings

Dysplasia
Carcinoma in situ
Invasive cancer of the vagina or cervix
Cervical infection

notes

computed tomography of the abdomen/chest (CT scan of the abdomen/chest, CAT scan of the abdomen/chest)

C

Type of test X-ray with contrast dye

Normal findings No evidence of abnormality

Test explanation

CT scan of the abdomen is a noninvasive, yet very accurate, x-ray procedure used to diagnose pathologic conditions such as tumors, cysts, abscesses, inflammation, perforation, bleeding, obstruction, aneurysms, and calculi of the abdominal and retroperitoneal organs.

CT of the chest is helpful in evaluating the thoracic organs for pathologic conditions such as tumors, nodules, hematomas, parenchymal coin lesions, cysts, abscesses, pleural effusion, and enlarged lymph nodes affecting the lungs and mediastinum. Tumors, cysts, and fractures of the chest wall and pleura can also be seen. When an IV contrast material is given, vascular structures can be identified, and a diagnosis of aortic or other vascular abnormalities can be made. With oral contrast, the esophagus and upper structures can be evaluated for tumors and other conditions.

Liver tumors, abscesses, trauma, cysts, and anatomic abnormalities can be seen, and pancreatic tumors, pseudocysts, inflammation, calcification, bleeding, and trauma can be detected.

The kidneys and urinary outflow tract are well visualized. Renal tumors and cysts, ureteral obstruction, calculi, and congenital renal and ureteral abnormalities are easily seen with the use of IV contrast injection. Extravasation of urine secondary to trauma or obstruction can also be demonstrated easily. Adrenal tumors and hyperplasia are best diagnosed with this technique.

Perforations of the bowel can be identified with the CT scan, especially when oral contrast is ingested. The spleen can be well visualized for hematoma, laceration, fracture, tumor infiltration, and splenic vein thrombosis with CT scanning. The retroperitoneal lymph nodes can be evaluated. The abdominal aorta and its major branches can be evaluated for aneurysmal dilation and intramural thrombi, and the pelvic structures (including the uterus, ovaries, tubes, prostate, and rectum) and musculature can be evaluated for tumors, abscesses, infection, or hypertrophy. Ascites and hemoperitoneum can easily be demonstrated with CT scan.

CT scan can also be used to guide aspiration of fluid from the abdomen or one of the abdominal organs. This fluid can be sent for cultures and other studies. The CT scan can also be used to guide biopsy needles into areas of abdominal or lung tumors to obtain tissues for study. Catheters for drainage of intraabdominal abscess can be placed with CT guidance.

CT scan is an important part of staging and monitoring of many tumors before and after therapy. Tumors of the mediastinum, colon, rectum, liver, breast, lung, prostate, ovary, uterus, kidney, lymph and adrenal glands commonly recur in the abdomen. Recurrence can be detected early with a CT scan.

Contraindications

- Patients who are allergic to iodinated dye or shellfish
- Patients who are pregnant
- Patients who are very obese, usually over 300 pounds

Potential complications

- Allergic reaction to iodinated dye
- Acute renal failure from dye infusion (adequate hydration before the infusion may reduce this likelihood)
- Hypoglycemia or acidosis may occur in patients who are taking Glucophage and who receive iodine dye.

Interfering factors

- Presence of metallic objects (e.g., hemostasis clips)
- Retained barium from previous studies

Procedure and patient care

Before

- Obtain informed consent if required by the institution.
- Assess the patient for allergies to iodinated dye or shellfish.
- Keep the patient NPO for at least 4 hours before the test if oral contrast is to be administered; however, this test can be performed on an emergency basis on patients who have recently eaten.

During

- Note the following procedure for the CT scan:
  1. The patient is taken to the radiology department and placed on the CT scan table.
  2. The patient is asked to remain motionless in a supine position because any motion will cause blurring and streaking of the final picture.

3. Through audio communication, the patient is instructed to hold his or her breath during x-ray exposure.
- Oral and IV iodinated x-ray contrast dye provides better results for this test.

After

- Encourage the patient to drink fluids to avoid dye-induced renal failure and to promote dye excretion.
- Inform the patient that diarrhea may occur after ingestion of the oral contrast.

Abnormal findings

Liver

Tumor   Bile duct dilation
Abscess

Pancreas

Tumor   Inflammation
Pseudocyst   Bleeding

Spleen

Hematoma   Tumor
Fracture   Venous thrombosis
Laceration

Gallbladder/biliary system

Gallstones   Bile duct dilation
Tumor

Kidneys

Tumor   Calculi
Cyst   Congenital abnormalities
Ureteral obstruction

Adrenal gland

Adenoma   Hemorrhage
Cancer   Myelolipoma hyperplasia
Pheochromocytoma

GI tract

Perforation   Diverticulitis
Tumor   Appendicitis
Inflammatory bowel
  disease

Uterus, tubes, ovaries

Tumor   Hydrosalpinx
Abscess   Cyst
Infection   Fibroid

Prostate

Hypertrophy   Tumor

Retroperitoneum

Tumor   Lymphadenopathy

Chest

Pulmonary tumor/nodules   Hiatal hernia
Pulmonary cyst   Mediastinal tumor (e.g.,
Pleural effusion   lymphoma, thymoma)
Pneumonitis   Primary or metastatic chest
Esophageal tumor   wall tumor

Other

Abdominal aneurysm
Ascites, hemoperitoneum
Abscess

notes

computed tomography of the brain (CT scan of the brain, Computerized axial transverse tomography [CATT])

Type of test X-ray with contrast dye

Normal findings No evidence of pathologic conditions

Test explanation

   CT scan of the brain is used in the differential diagnosis of intracranial neoplasms, cerebral infarctions, ventricular displacement or enlargement, cortical atrophy, cerebral aneurysms, intracranial hemorrhage and hematoma, and arteriovenous (AV) malformation. Information about the ventricular system can also be obtained by CT scanning. Multiple sclerosis and other degenerative abnormalities can be identified also.

   Visualization of a neoplasm, previous infarction, or any pathologic process that destroys the blood-brain barrier may be enhanced by IV injection of an iodinated contrast dye. CT scans may be repeated to monitor the progress of any disease or to monitor the healing process. In many localities, MRI scanning of the brain has replaced the use of CT scans of the brain.

Contraindications See p. 87, CT scan of abdomen and chest.

Potential complications See p. 87, CT scan of abdomen and chest.

Procedure and patient care

Before

- Obtain informed consent if required by the institution.
- Keep the patient NPO for 4 hours before the study because contrast dye may cause nausea.
- Instruct the patient that wigs, hairpins, clips, or partial dental plates cannot be worn during the procedure because they hamper visualization of the brain.
- Assess the patient for allergies to iodinated dye or shellfish.

During

- Note the following procedure for the brain CT scan.
  1. The patient lies in the supine position on an examining table with the head resting on a snug-fitting rubber cap within a water-filled box.

2. The patient's head is enclosed only to the hairline (as in a hair dryer). The face is not covered, and the patient can see out of the machine at all times.
3. Sponges are placed along the side of the head to ensure that the patient's head does not move during the study.
4. An iodinated dye will usually then be used. A peripheral IV line is started, and the iodine dye is administered through it.
5. The entire scanning process is repeated.

After

- Encourage the patient to drink fluids because dye is excreted by the kidneys and causes diuresis.

Abnormal findings

Intracranial neoplasm
Cerebral infarction
Ventricular displacement
Ventricular enlargement
Cortical atrophy
Cerebral aneurysm
Intracranial hemorrhage

Hematoma
AV malformation
Meningioma
Multiple sclerosis
Hydrocephalus
Abscess

notes

COOMBS' TESTING

Coombs' test, direct (Direct antiglobulin test)
Coombs' test, indirect (Blood antibody screening)

Type of test Blood

Normal findings Negative; no agglutination

Test explanation

The Coombs' test is performed to identify immune-mediated hemolysis (destruction of RBCs) or to investigate hemolytic transfusion reactions. The *direct Coombs' test* demonstrates if the patient's (or transfused) RBCs have been attacked by antibodies in the patient's own bloodstream.

The *indirect Coombs' test* detects circulating antibodies against RBCs. The major purpose of the test is to determine if the patient has minor serum antibodies (other than the major ABO/Rh system) to RBCs that he or she is about to receive by blood transfusion. Therefore this test is the "screening" part of the "type and screen" routinely performed for blood compatibility testing (crossmatching in the blood bank). This test is also used to detect other agglutinins such as cold agglutinins, which are associated with mycoplasmal infections.

Coombs' serum is a solution containing antibodies to human globulin (antibodies). The direct Coombs' test is performed on the patient's RBCs. The indirect Coombs's test is performed on the patient's serum.

In the direct Coombs' test, Coombs' serum is mixed with the patient's RBCs. If the RBCs have antibodies on them, agglutination of the patient's RBCs will occur. The greater the quantity of antibodies against RBCs, the more clumping occurs. This test is read as *positive,* with clumping on a scale of trace to +4. If the RBCs are not coated with autoantibodies against RBCs (immunoglobulins), agglutination will not occur; this is a *negative* test.

In the indirect Coombs' test, a small amount of the recipient's serum is added to donor RBCs containing known antibodies on their surface. This is the first stage. In the second stage of the test, Coombs' serum is added. Coombs' serum is a solution containing antibodies to human globulin (antibodies). If antibodies exist in the patient's serum, agglutination occurs. In blood transfusion screening, visible agglutination indicates that the recipient has antibodies to the donor's RBCs.

Interfering factors

☛ Drugs that may cause false-positive results include ampicillin, captopril, cephalosporins, chlorpromazine (Thorazine), insulin, isoniazid (INH), levodopa, phenytoin (Dilantin), procainamide, quinidine, rifampin, and sulfonamides.

Procedure and patient care

Before
- Tell the patient that no fasting is required.

During
- Collect approximately 5 to 7 ml of venous blood in a red- or lavender-top tube.

After
- Apply pressure to the venipuncture site.

Abnormal findings

Autoimmune hemolytic anemia
Transfusion reaction
Erythroblastosis fetalis
Lymphoma
Lupus erythematosus
Mycoplasmal infection
Infectious mononucleosis
Presence of specific cold agglutinin antibody

notes

creatine phosphokinase (CPK, CP, Creatine kinase [CK])

Type of test Blood

Normal findings

Total CPK

Adult/elderly
    Male: 12-70 U/ml or 55-170 U/L (SI units)
    Female: 10-55 U/ml or 30-135 U/L (SI units)
Values are higher after exercise.
Newborn: 68-580 U/L (SI units)

Isoenzymes

CPK-MM: 100%
CPK-MB: 0%
CPK-BB: 0%

Test explanation

CPK is found predominantly in the heart muscle, skeletal muscle, and brain. Serum CPK levels are elevated whenever injury occurs to these muscle or nerve cells. CPK levels can rise within 6 hours after damage. If damage is not persistent, the levels peak at 18 hours after injury and return to normal in 2 to 3 days.

To test specifically for myocardial muscle injury, electrophoresis is performed to detect the three *CPK isoenzymes:* CPK-BB (CPK1), CPK-MB (CPK2), and CPK-MM (CPK3). The CPK-MB isoenzyme part appears to be specific for myocardial cells. CPK-MB levels rise 3 to 6 hours after infarction occurs. If there is no further myocardial damage, the level peaks at 12 to 24 hours and returns to normal 12 to 48 hours after infarction. CPK-MB levels do not usually rise with transient chest pain caused by angina, pulmonary embolism, or congestive heart failure. One can expect to see a rise in CPK-MB in patients with unstable angina, shock, malignant hyperthermia, myopathies, or myocarditis. Very small amounts of CPK-MB also exist in skeletal muscle. Severe injury to skeletal muscle can be significant enough to raise the CPK-MB isoenzyme above normal. To avoid the misdiagnosis of myocardial injury, a *relative index* is calculated to determine whether myocardial injury has occurred. This relative index is a mathematic calculation of the ratio of CPK-MB to total CPK. A relative index of >2.5 is highly suggestive of myocardial injury.

The CPK-MB isoenzyme level is helpful in both quantifying the degree of myocardial infarction and timing the onset of infarction. With the more frequent use of thrombolytic therapy for myocardial infarction, the CPK-MB isoenzyme is often used to determine appropriateness of thrombolytic therapy. High CPK-MB levels would suggest that significant infarction has already occurred, thereby precluding the benefit of thrombolytic therapy.

Because the CPK-BB isoenzyme is predominantly found in the brain and lung, injury to either of these organs (e.g., cerebrovascular accident, pulmonary infarction) is associated with elevated levels of this isoenzyme.

When the CPK-MM level is elevated, injury to or disease of the skeletal muscle is present. Examples of this include myopathies, vigorous exercise, multiple IM injections, electroconvulsive therapy, chronic alcoholism, or surgery.

Each isoenzyme has been found to have isoforms. The CPK-MM isoforms MM1 and MM3 are most useful for cardiac disease. A MM3/MM1 ratio of greater than 1 suggests acute myocardial injury. The CPK-MB ratio of MB2/MB1 isoforms greater than 1 also indicates acute myocardial injury.

Interfering factors

- IM injections can cause elevated CPK levels.
- Strenuous exercise and recent surgery may cause increased levels.

Procedure and patient care

Before

- Discuss with the patient the need and reason for frequent venipuncture in diagnosing myocardial infarction.
- Avoid IM injections in patients with cardiac disease. These injections may falsely elevate the total CPK level.
- Tell the patient that no food or fluid restrictions are necessary.

During

- Collect a venous blood sample in a red-top tube. This is usually done daily for 3 days and then at 1 week.
- Rotate the venipuncture sites.
- Avoid hemolysis.
- Record the exact time and date of venipuncture on each laboratory slip. This aids in the interpretation of the temporal pattern of enzyme elevations.

After
- Apply pressure to the venipuncture site.

Abnormal findings

▲ **Increased levels of total CPK**
Diseases or injury affecting the heart muscle, skeletal muscle, and brain

▲ **Increased levels of CPK-BB isoenzyme**
Diseases affecting the central nervous system
Adenocarcinoma (especially breast and lung)
Pulmonary infarction

▲ **Increased levels of CPK-MB isoenzyme**
Acute myocardial infarction
Cardiac aneurysm surgery
Cardiac defibrillation
Myocarditis
Ventricular arrhythmias
Cardiac ischemia

▲ **Increased levels of CPK-MM isoenzyme**
Rhabdomyolysis
Muscular dystrophy
Myositis
Recent surgery
Electromyography
IM injections
Crush injuries
Delirium tremens
Malignant hyperthermia
Recent convulsions
Electroconvulsive therapy
Shock
Hypokalemia
Hypothyroidism

notes

creatinine, blood (Serum creatinine)

Type of test Blood

Normal findings

Adult

   Female: 0.5-1.1 mg/dl or 44-97 μmol/L (SI units)
   Male: 0.6-1.2 mg/dl
Elderly: decrease in muscle mass may cause decreased values
Adolescent: 0.5-1.0 mg/dl
Child: 0.3-0.7 mg/dl
Infant: 0.2-0.4 mg/dl
Newborn: 0.3-1.2 mg/dl

Possible critical values >4 mg/dl (indicates serious impairment in renal function)

Test explanation

   This test measures the amount of creatinine in the blood. Creatinine is a catabolic product of creatine phosphate, which is used in skeletal muscle contraction. The daily production of creatine, and subsequently creatinine, depends on muscle mass, which fluctuates very little. Creatinine, as with blood urea nitrogen (BUN, see p. 280), is excreted entirely by the kidneys and therefore is directly proportional to renal excretory function. Thus, with normal renal excretory function, the serum creatinine level should remain constant and normal. Only renal disorders such as glomerulonephritis, pyelonephritis, acute tubular necrosis, and urinary obstruction, will cause an abnormal elevation in creatinine.

   The serum creatinine test, as with the BUN, is used to diagnose impaired renal function. In general, a doubling of creatinine suggests a 50% reduction in the glomerular filtration rate. The creatinine level is interpreted in conjunction with the BUN. These tests are referred to as *renal function studies*.

Interfering factors

☞ Drugs that may *increase* creatinine values include aminoglycosides (e.g., gentamicin), heavy-metal chemotherapeutic agents (e.g., cisplatin), and other nephrotoxic drugs.

Procedure and patient care

Before
- Tell the patient that no fasting is required.

During
- Collect approximately 5 ml of blood in a red-top tube.
- For pediatric patients, blood is usually drawn from a heel stick.

After
- Apply pressure to the venipuncture site.

Abnormal findings

▲ **Increased levels**
Glomerulonephritis
Pyelonephritis
Acute tubular necrosis
Urinary tract obstruction
Reduced renal blood flow
  (e.g., shock, dehydra-
  tion, congestive heart
  failure, atherosclerosis)
Diabetic nephropathy
Nephritis
Rhabdomyolysis
Acromegaly
Gigantism

▼ **Decreased levels**
Debilitation
Decreased muscle mass
  (e.g., muscular dystro-
  phy, myasthenia gravis)

notes

creatinine clearance (CC)

Type of test   Urine (24-hour); blood

Normal findings
<Adult (40 years)
  Male: 90-139 ml/min or 0.87-1.34 ml/sec/m²
  Female: 80-125 ml/min or 0.77-1.20 ml/sec/m²
Values decrease 6.5 ml/min/decade of life because of decline
  in glomerular filtration rate (GFR).
Newborn: 40-65 ml/min

Test explanation
  Creatinine is a catabolic product of creatine phosphate, which
is used in skeletal muscle contraction. The daily production of
creatinine depends on muscle mass, which fluctuates very little.
Creatinine is entirely excreted by the kidneys and therefore is directly proportional to the glomerular filtration rate (GFR; i.e.,
the number of milliliters of filtrate made by the kidneys per
minute). The creatinine clearance (CC) is a measure of the glomerular filtration rate.
  The CC depends on the amount of blood present to be filtered
and the ability of the glomeruli to act as a filter. The amount of
blood present for filtration is decreased in renal artery atherosclerosis, dehydration, or shock. The ability of the glomeruli to act as
a filter is decreased by diseases such as glomerulonephritis, acute
tubular necrosis, and most other primary renal diseases. The CC
is reduced in these diseases.
  When one kidney alone becomes diseased, the opposite kidney,
if normal, has the ability to compensate by increasing its filtration
rate. Therefore, with unilateral kidney disease or nephrectomy, a
decrease in CC is not expected if the other kidney is normal.
  The CC test requires a 24-hour urine collection and a serum
creatinine level. Creatinine clearance is then computed using the
following formula:

$$\text{Creatinine clearance} = \frac{UV}{P}$$

  where
U = Number of milligrams per deciliter of creatinine excreted
  in the urine over 24 hours

V = Volume of urine in milliliters per minute
P = Serum creatinine in milligrams per deciliter

A 24-hour urine collection for creatinine is often measured along with other urine collections to assess the completeness of other 24-hour collections. In patients with normal creatinine, the CC should indicate whether all the urine has been collected for the 24 hours.

Interfering factors

- Exercise may cause increased creatinine values.
- Incomplete urine collection may give a falsely lowered value.
- A diet high in meat content can transiently cause elevation of the creatinine clearance.
- Drugs that may cause *increased* levels include aminoglycosides (e.g., gentamicin), heavy-metal chemotherapeutic agents (e.g., cisplatin), and nephrotoxic drugs.

Procedure and patient care

Before

- Tell the patient that no special diet is usually required.
- Note that some laboratories instruct the patient to avoid cooked meat, tea, coffee, or drugs on the day of the test. Check with the laboratory.

During

- Instruct the patient to begin the 24-hour urine collection after voiding. Discard the initial specimen and start the 24-hour timing as of that point.
- Collect all the urine passed during the next 24 hours.
- Show the patient where to store the urine specimen.
- Keep the specimen on ice or refrigerated during the 24 hours.
- Post the hours for the urine collection in a noticeable place to prevent accidental discharge of a specimen.
- Instruct the patient to void before defecating so that urine is not contaminated by feces.
- Remind the patient not to put toilet paper in the collection container.
- Encourage the patient to drink fluids during the 24 hours unless this is contraindicated for medical purposes.
- Instruct the patient to avoid vigorous exercise during the 24 hours because exercise may cause an increased creatinine clearance.

- Make sure a venous blood sample is drawn in a red-top tube during the 24-hour collection.
- Mark the patient's age, weight, and height on the requisition sheet.

After

- Transport the urine specimen promptly to the laboratory.
- Apply pressure to the venipuncture site.

Abnormal findings

▲ **Increased levels**
Exercise
Pregnancy
High cardiac output syndromes

▼ **Decreased levels**
Impaired kidney function (e.g., renal artery atherosclerosis, glomerulonephritis, acute tubular necrosis)
Conditions causing decreased GFR (e.g., congestive heart failure, cirrhosis with ascites, shock, dehydration)

notes

CULTURE AND SENSITIVITY (C & S)
wound culture and sensitivity
urine culture and sensitivity
throat culture and sensitivity
sputum culture and sensitivity
blood culture and sensitivity

Type of test Microscopic examination

Normal findings
No growth after 72 hours

Urine:
Negative: fewer than 10,000 bacteria/ml of urine
Positive: greater than 100,000 bacteria/ml of urine

Test explanation
Cultures are obtained to determine the presence of pathogens in patients with suspected infections. All cultures should be performed before antibiotic therapy is initiated. Otherwise, the antibiotic may interrupt the growth of the organism in the laboratory. If the patient is receiving antibiotics during the time that the culture is obtained, resin can be added to the culture medium to negate the antibiotic effect of inhibiting growth of the offending bacteria in the culture.

An important part of any routine culture is to assess the sensitivity of any bacteria that is growing to various antibiotics. The physician can then more appropriately recommend the correct antibiotic therapy. Antibiotics that are safest, least expensive, and most effective for treatment of that specific bacteria are prescribed.

More often than not, however, the physician will want to institute antibiotic therapy before the culture results are reported. In these instances, a *Gram stain* of the specimen smeared on a slide is most helpful and can be reported in less than 10 minutes. All forms of bacteria are grossly classified as gram positive (blue staining) or gram negative (red staining). Knowledge of the shape of the organism (e.g., spheric, rod shaped) may also be very helpful in the tentative identification of the infecting organism. Most organisms require approximately 24 hours to grow in the laboratory, and a preliminary report can be given at that time. Occasionally 48 to 72 hours are required for growth and identification of the organism. Cultures may be repeated after appropriate antibiotic therapy to assess for complete resolution of the infection.

Wound infections are most often caused by pus-forming organisms. The exudate or pus is cultured.

Urine cultures and sensitivities are obtained to determine the presence of urinary tract infections involving the kidneys, ureters, bladder, or urethra. To preserve resources, urine cultures are done only if the urinalysis suggests a possible infection (e.g., increased number of white blood cells [WBCs], bacteria, high pH, positive leukocyte esterase). The urine is collected and "split." One half is sent for urinalysis, and the other half is held in the laboratory refrigerator and evaluated only if the urinalysis indicates a possible infection.

Because the throat is normally colonized by many organisms, culture of this area serves only to isolate and identify a few particular pathogens (e.g., streptococci, meningococci, gonococci, *Bordetella pertussis, Corynebacterium diphtheriae*). Recognition of these organisms requires treatment. Streptococci are most often sought because a beta-hemolytic streptococcal pharyngitis may be followed by rheumatic heart disease or glomerulonephritis. Rapid immunologic tests *(strept screen)* with antiserum against group A streptococcus antigen are now available and are very accurate. These tests can be performed in about 15 minutes.

Sputum cultures are obtained to determine the presence of pathogenic bacteria in patients with respiratory infections, such as bronchitis or pneumonia. Sputum cultures for fungus and *Mycobacterium tuberculosis* may take 6 to 8 weeks.

Blood cultures are obtained to detect the presence of bacteria in the blood. Bacteremia (the presence of bacteria in the blood) can be intermittent and transient. The episode of bacteremia is usually accompanied by chills and fever; thus the blood culture should be drawn when the patient manifests these signs to increase the chances of growing out bacteria on the cultures. It is important that at least two culture specimens be obtained from two different sites. If one produces bacteria and the other does not, it is safe to assume that the bacteria in the first culture may be a contaminant and not the infecting agent. If cultures are to be performed while the patient is on antibiotics, the blood culture specimen should be taken shortly before the next dose of the antibiotic is administered.

Culture specimens drawn through an IV catheter are frequently contaminated, and tests using them should not be performed unless catheter sepsis is suspected.

Interfering factors

- Drugs that may alter test results include antibiotics.
- Mouthwash may alter throat cultures.
- Contamination of the urine with stool or vaginal secretions will cause false positives.

Procedure and patient care

Before
- For sputum culture:
  1. Remind the patient that sputum must be coughed up from the lungs and that saliva is not sputum.
  2. Instruct the patient to rinse out his or her mouth with water before the sputum collection to decrease contamination of the sputum by particles in the oropharynx.

During
- Handle all specimens as though they were capable of transmitting disease.
- For wound culture:
  1. Aseptically place a sterile cotton swab into the pus of the patient's wound and then place the swab into a sterile, covered test tube.
  2. If any antibiotic ointment or solution has been previously applied, remove it with sterile water or saline before obtaining the culture.
- For urine culture:
  1. A *clean-catch* or *midstream urine* collection is required for C & S testing. This requires meticulous cleansing of the urinary meatus with an iodine preparation to reduce contamination. Then the cleansing agent must be completely removed or it will contaminate the urine specimen. The midstream collection is obtained by:
     a. Having the patient begin to urinate in a bedpan, urinal, or toilet and then stop urinating (this washes the urine out of the distal urethra)
     b. Correctly positioning a sterile urine container into which the patient voids 3 to 4 ounces of urine
     c. Capping the container
     d. Allowing the patient to finish voiding
  2. Note that *urinary catheterization* may be needed for patients unable to void. For inpatients who already have an *indwelling urinary catheter,* obtain a specimen by attaching a small-gauge (e.g., No. 25) needle to a syringe and

aseptically inserting the needle into the catheter at a point distal to the sleeve leading to the balloon. Urine is aspirated and then placed in a sterile urine container. *Suprapubic aspiration* of urine is a safe method of obtaining urine in neonates and infants. The abdomen is prepared with an antiseptic, and a 25-gauge needle is inserted into the suprapubic area 1 inch above the symphysis pubis. Urine is aspirated into the syringe and then transferred to a sterile urine container.

3. Collect specimens from infants and young children in a disposable pouch called a *U bag*. This bag has an adhesive backing around the opening to attach to the child.

- For throat culture:
    1. Obtain a throat culture by depressing the tongue with a wooden tongue blade and touching the posterior wall of the throat and areas of inflammation, exudation, or ulceration with a sterile cotton swab.
    2. Avoid touching any other part of the mouth.
- For sputum culture:
    1. Note that sputum specimens are best when the patient awakens in the morning before eating or drinking.
    2. Collect at least 1 teaspoon of sputum in a sterile sputum container.
    3. Usually obtain sputum by having the patient cough after taking several deep breaths.
    4. If the patient is unable to produce a sputum specimen, stimulate coughing by lowering the head of the patient's bed or giving the patient an aerosol administration of a warm, hypertonic solution.
    5. Note that other methods to collect sputum include endotracheal aspiration, fiberoptic bronchoscopy, and transtracheal aspiration.
- For blood culture:
    1. Carefully prepare the proposed venipuncture site with povidone-iodine (Betadine). Allow the skin to dry.
    2. Clean the tops of the Vacutainer tubes or culture bottles with povidone-iodine and allow them to dry. Some laboratories suggest cleaning with 70% alcohol after cleaning with povidone-iodine and air drying.
    3. Collect approximately 10 to 15 ml of venous blood by venipuncture from each site in a 20-ml syringe.

4. Discard the needle on the syringe and replace with a second sterile needle before injecting the blood sample into the culture bottle.
5. Inoculate the anaerobic bottle first if both anaerobic and aerobic cultures are needed.
6. Mix gently after inoculation.

After
- Label the specimen with the patient's name, date, time, and tentative diagnosis.
- Transport the specimen to the laboratory immediately after testing (at least within 30 minutes).
- Notify the physician of any positive results so that appropriate antibiotic therapy can be initiated.

Abnormal findings

Wound infection
Urinary tract infection
Pharyngitis
Bacteremia

Pneumonia
Bronchitis
Atypical pneumonia (e.g., tuberculosis)

notes

cystoscopy (Endourology)

Type of test Endoscopy

Normal findings Normal structure and function of the urethra, bladder, ureters, and prostate (in males)

Test explanation

Cystoscopy provides direct visualization of the urethra and bladder through the transurethral insertion of a cystoscope into the bladder. Cystoscopy is used *diagnostically* to allow:

1. Direct inspection and biopsy of the prostate, bladder, and urethra
2. Collection of a separate urine specimen directly from each kidney by the placement of ureteral catheters
3. Measurement of bladder capacity and determination of ureteral reflux
4. Identification of bladder and ureteral calculi
5. Placement of ureteral catheters for retrograde pyelography
6. Identification of the source of hematuria

Cystoscopy is used *therapeutically* to provide:

1. Resection of small, superficial bladder tumors
2. Removal of foreign bodies and stones
3. Coagulation of bleeding areas
4. Implantation of radium seeds into a tumor
5. Resection of hypertrophied or malignant prostate gland overgrowth
6. Placement of ureteral stents for identification of ureters during pelvic surgery

Cystoscopy is important in the evaluation of hematuria, chronic infection, suspected stones, and radiographic filling defects. On inspection, the urethra may show inflammation or structural causes of obstruction (e.g., stricture, neoplasia, prostatic hypertrophy). If the obstruction is functional rather than structural (e.g., detrusor-bladder neck dyssynergia), no site of obstruction will be demonstrated by endoscopy.

Potential complications

- Perforation of the bladder
- Sepsis by seeding the bloodstream with bacteria from infected urine

- Hematuria
- Urinary retention

Procedure and patient care

Before

- Ensure that an informed consent is obtained.
- If enemas are ordered to clear the bowel, assist the patient as needed and record the results.
- Encourage the patient to drink fluids several hours before the procedure to maintain a continuous flow of urine for collection and to prevent multiplication of bacteria that may be introduced during this technique.
- If the procedure will be performed with the patient under general anesthesia, follow routine precautions. Keep the patient NPO after midnight on the day of the test. Fluids may be given intravenously.

During

- Cleanse the external genitalia with an antiseptic solution such as povidone-iodine (Betadine), (the cystoscope is inserted, and the desired diagnostic or therapeutic studies are performed).
- Tell the patient that he or she will have the desire to void as the cystoscope passes the bladder neck.
- When the procedure is completed, keep the patient on bed rest for a short time.
- Note that this procedure is performed by a urologist in approximately 25 minutes.
- When local anesthesia is used, inform the patient of the associated discomfort (much more than with urethral catheterization).

After

- Assess the patient's ability to void for at least 24 hours after the procedure. Urinary retention may be secondary to edema caused by instrumentation.
- Note the urine color. Pink-tinged urine is common. The presence of bright-red blood or clots should be reported to the physician.
- Encourage increased intake of fluids. A dilute urine decreases dysuria. Fluids also maintain a constant flow of urine to prevent stasis and the accumulation of bacteria in the bladder.

- Observe for signs and symptoms of sepsis (elevated temperature, flush, chills, decreased blood pressure, increased pulse).
- Note that antibiotics are occasionally ordered 1 day before and 3 days following the procedure to reduce the incidence of bacteremia that may occur with instrumentation of the urethra and bladder.
- Encourage the patient to use cathartics, especially after cystoscopic surgery. Increases in intraabdominal pressure caused by constipation may initiate severe lower urologic bleeding.
- If postprocedure irrigation is ordered, have the patient use an isotonic solution containing mannitol, glycine, or sorbitol to prevent fluid overhydration in the event any of the irrigation is absorbed through opened venous sinuses in the bladder.
- If a catheter is left in after the procedure, provide catheter care instructions.

Abnormal findings

Lower urologic tract tumor
Stones in the ureter or bladder
Prostatic hypertrophy
Prostate cancer
Inflammation of the bladder and urethra
Urethral/ureteral stricture
Prostatitis
Vesical neck contracture

notes

Doppler studies, vascular

Type of test Ultrasound

Normal findings

Venous

A normal Doppler venous signal with spontaneous respiration
Normal venous system without evidence of occlusion

Arterial

Normal arterial Doppler signal with systolic and diastolic components

No reduction in blood pressure in excess of 20 mm Hg compared with the normal extremity

A normal ankle-to-brachial arterial blood pressure index of 0.85 or greater

No evidence of arterial occlusion

Test explanation

Doppler studies are used to identify occlusion of the veins or arteries. Although this discussion is limited to the extremities, this technology is also performed on the carotid artery (see p. 76) and on the arterial system of the viscera (e.g., liver, kidney and bowel.) In the extremity, arterial Doppler studies are used on patients with suspected arterial insufficiency (such as claudication, poorly healing skin ulcer, cold pale leg, pulseless extremity, or rest pain). Venous ultrasound is used to evaluate the patency of the venous system in patients with a swollen painful leg, venous varicosities of the upper or lower extremity, or an edematous extremity. Venous doppler studies are not accurate for venous occlusive disease of the lower calf.

With *arterial* Doppler studies, one can identify and locate peripheral arteriosclerotic occlusive disease of the extremities. This can be done with a single mode ultrasound by slowly deflating blood pressure cuffs placed on the thigh, calf, and ankle. The systolic pressure in the various arteries of the extremities can be accurately measured by detecting the first evidence of blood flow with the Doppler transducer. The extremely sensitive Doppler ultrasound detector can recognize the "swishing" sound of even the most minimal blood flow. Normally there is a minimal drop in systolic blood pressure from the arteries of the arms to those of the legs. If the drop in blood pressure exceeds 20 mm Hg, occlusive disease is believed to exist immediately proximal to the area tested.

With a duplex mode ultrasound, a two-dimensional image of the artery can be produced. As a result, one can directly visualize possibly stenotic or occluded arteries and arterial flow disruption. Lower extremity arterial bypass graft patency can also be assessed by Doppler ultrasound.

Interfering factors

- Venous or arterial occlusive disease proximal to the site of testing
- Cigarette smoking because nicotine can cause constriction of the peripheral arteries and alter the results

Procedure and patient care

Before

- Remove all clothing from the extremity to be examined.
- Instruct the patient to abstain from cigarette smoking for at least 30 minutes before the test.

During

- Note the following procedural steps:

  Venous Doppler studies
  1. A conductive gel is applied to the skin overlying the venous system of the extremity in multiple areas.
  2. Usually, for the lower extremity, the deep venous system is identified in the ankle, calf, thigh, and groin.
  3. The characteristic "swishing" sound of the Doppler indicates a patent venous system. Failure to detect this signal indicates venous occlusion.
  4. Usually both the superficial and deep venous systems are evaluated.

  Arterial Doppler studies
  1. These are performed with the use of blood pressure cuffs, which are placed around the thigh, calf, and ankle.
  2. A conductive paste is applied to the skin overlying the artery distal to the cuffs.
  3. The proximal cuff is inflated to a level above systolic blood pressure in the normal extremity.
  4. The Doppler ultrasound transducer is placed immediately distal to the inflated cuff.
  5. The pressure in the cuff is slowly released.
  6. The highest pressure at which blood flow is detected by

the characteristic "swishing" Doppler signal is recorded as the blood pressure of that artery.

7. The test is repeated at each successive level.
8. When the ankle pressure is divided by the arm (brachial artery) pressure, this is known as the AB index. If the *AB index* is less than 0.85, significant arterial occlusive disease exists within the extremity.

- Note that these studies are usually performed in the vascular laboratory or radiology department and take approximately 30 minutes.
- Duplex scanning is then performed visualizing the vessels in question.

After

- Remove the transducer gel from the extremity.

Abnormal findings

Venous occlusion, secondary to thrombosis or thrombophlebitis
Venous varicosities
Small or large vessel arterial occlusive disease
Spastic arterial disease (e.g., Raynaud's phenomenon)
Small vessel arterial occlusive disease (as in diabetes)
Embolic arterial occlusion
Arterial aneurysm

notes

echocardiography (Cardiac echo, Heart sonogram, Transthoracic echocardiography [TTE])

Type of test   Ultrasound

Normal findings

Normal position, size, and movement of the cardiac valves and heart muscle wall
Normal directional flow of blood within the heart chambers

Test explanation

Echocardiography is a noninvasive ultrasound procedure used to evaluate the structure and function of the heart. The study usually includes M-mode recordings, two-dimensional recordings, and a Doppler study.

M-mode echocardiography is a linear tracing of the motion of the heart structures over time. This allows the various cardiac structures to be located and studied regarding their movement during a cardiac cycle.

Two-dimensional echocardiography angles a beam within one sector of the heart. This produces a picture of the spatial anatomic relationships within the heart.

A recent addition has been *color Doppler echocardiography.* This test detects the pattern of the blood flow and measures changes in velocity of blood flow within the heart and great vessels. Turbulent blood or altered velocity and direction of blood flow can be identified by changes in color. The most useful application of the color flow imaging is in determining the direction and turbulence of blood flow across regurgitant or narrowed valves.

Echocardiography, in general, is used in the diagnosis of pericardial effusion, valvular heart disease (e.g., mitral valve prolapse, stenosis, regurgitation), subaortic stenosis, myocardial wall abnormalities (e.g., cardiomyopathy), infarction, or aneurysm. Cardiac tumors (e.g., myxomas) are easily diagnosed with ultrasound. Atrial and ventricular septal defects and other congenital heart diseases are also recognized by ultrasound. Finally, postinfarction mural thrombi are readily apparent with this testing.

Echocardiography is also used in *cardiac stress testing.* It is fast becoming the method of choice in heart imaging for stress testing. During an exercise or chemical cardiac stress test, ischemic muscle areas are evident as hypokinetic areas within the myocardium. Echocardiography is being used with increased frequency in emergent and urgent evaluations of patients with chest pains. If the myocardium is normal and without areas of hypokinesia, no coronary artery occlusive disease is suspected. If, however a hypokinetic or akinetic area is noted, ischemia or infarction has occurred, and the chest pain is cardiac in origin.

It is now possible to perform echocardiography via the esophagus using a probe mounted on an endoscope. This is referred to as *transesophageal echocardiography, TEE.*

Contraindications

- Patients who are uncooperative

Interfering factors

- Chronic obstructive pulmonary disease (COPD).
  Patients who have severe COPD have a significant amount of air and space between the heart and the chest cavity. Air space does not conduct ultrasound waves well.
- Obesity
  In obese patients the space between the heart and the transducer is greatly enlarged; therefore accuracy of the test is decreased.

Procedure and patient care

Before

- No special preparation is required.

During

- Note the following procedural steps:
  1. The patient is placed in the supine position.
  2. Electrocardiographic (ECG) leads are placed.
  3. A gel is placed on the chest wall immediately under the transducer.
  4. Ultrasound is directed to the heart, and appropriate tracings are obtained.
- Note that this procedure usually takes approximately 45 minutes and is performed by an ultrasound technician in a darkened room within the cardiac laboratory or radiology department.

After

- Remove the gel from the patient's chest wall.

Abnormal findings

Valvular stenosis
Valvular regurgitation
Mitral valve prolapse
Pericardial effusion
Ventricular or atrial
  mural thrombi

Myxoma
Poor ventricular muscle
  motion
Septal defects
Ventricular hypertrophy
Endocarditis

notes

electrocardiography (Electrocardiogram [ECG, EKG])

Type of test Electrodiagnostic

Normal findings Normal heart rate (60-100 beats/min), rhythm, and wave deflections

Test explanation

The ECG is a graphic representation of the electrical impulses that the heart generates during the cardiac cycle. These electrical impulses are conducted to the body's surface, where they are detected by electrodes placed on the patient's limbs and chest. The monitoring electrodes detect the electrical activity of the heart from a variety of spatial perspectives. The ECG lead system is composed of several electrodes that are placed on each of the four extremities and at varying sites on the chest. Each combination of electrodes is called a *lead*.

A *12-lead ECG* provides a comprehensive view of the flow of the heart's electrical currents in two different planes. There are six limb leads (combination of electrodes on the extremities) and six chest leads (corresponding to six sites on the chest). Leads I, II, and III are considered the standard *limb* leads. Lead I records the difference in electrical potential between the left arm (LA) and the right arm (RA). Lead II records the electrical potential between the RA and the left leg (LL). Lead III reflects the difference between the LA and the LL. The right leg (RL) electrode is an inactive ground in all leads. There are three *augmented* limb leads: aV_R, aV_L, and aV_F (*a*, augmented; *V*, vector [unipolar]; *R*, right arm; *L*, left arm; *F*, left foot or leg). The augmented leads measure the electrode potential between the center of the heart and the right arm (aV_R), the left arm (aV_L), and the left leg (aV_F). The six standard chest, or precordial, leads (V_1, V_2, V_3, V_4, V_5, V_6) are recorded by placing electrodes at six different positions on the chest, surrounding the heart.

In general, it is said that leads II, III and aV_F look at the inferior part of the heart. Leads aV_L and I look at the lateral part of the heart. Leads V_2-V_4 look at the anterior part of the heart.

The ECG is recorded on special paper with a graphic back of horizontal and vertical lines for rapid measurement of time intervals (*X* coordinate) and voltages (*Y* coordinate). Time duration is measured by vertical lines 1 mm apart, each representing 0.04

second. Voltage is measured by horizontal lines 1 mm apart. Five 1-mm squares equal 0.5 mV.

The normal ECG pattern is composed of waves arbitrarily designated by the letters *P, Q, R, S,* and *T.* The Q, R, and S waves are grouped together and are described as the QRS complex. The significance of the waves and time intervals is as follows.

P wave

This represents atrial electrical depolarization associated with atrial contraction.

PR interval

This represents the time required for the impulse to travel from the SA node to the atrioventricular (AV) node.

QRS complex

This represents ventricular electrical depolarization associated with ventricular contraction. This complex consists of an initial downward (negative) deflection (Q wave), a large upward (positive) deflection (R wave), and a small downward deflection (S wave).

ST segment

This represents the period between the completion of depolarization and the beginning of repolarization of the ventricular muscle. This segment may be elevated or depressed in transient muscle ischemia (e.g., angina) or in muscle injury (as in the early stages of myocardial infarction).

T wave

This represents ventricular repolarization (i.e., return to neutral electrical activity).

Through the analysis of these waveforms and time intervals, valuable information about the heart may be obtained. The ECG is used primarily to identify abnormal heart rhythms (arrhythmias [dysrhythmias]) and to diagnose acute myocardial infarction, conduction defects, and ventricular hypertrophy.

Interfering factors

- Inaccurate placement of the electrodes
- Electrolyte imbalances
- Poor contact between the skin and the electrodes
- Movement or muscle twitching during the test
- Drugs that can affect results include digitalis, quinidine, and barbiturates

Procedure and patient care

Before

- Tell the patient that no food or fluid restriction is necessary.

During

- Electrode paste is applied to ensure electrical conduction between the skin and the electrodes.
- The leads are applied to each arm and leg. The chest leads are positioned as follows:

  V_1: in the fourth intercostal space (4ICS) at the right sternal border

  V_2: in 4ICS at the left sternal border

  V_3: midway between V_2 and V_4

  V_4: in 5ICS at the midclavicular line

  V_5: at the left anterior axillary line at the level of V_4 horizontally

  V_6: at the left midaxillary line on the level of V_4 horizontally

After

- Remove the electrodes from the patient's skin and wipe off the electrode gel.

Abnormal findings

Arrhythmia
Acute myocardial infarction
Myocardial ischemia
Old myocardial infarction
Conduction defects
Conduction system disease
Wolff-Parkinson-White syndrome

Ventricular hypertrophy
Cor pulmonale
Pulmonary embolus
Electrolyte imbalance
Pericarditis

notes

endometrial biopsy

Type of test Microscopic examination of tissue

Normal findings

No pathologic conditions
Presence of a "secretory-type" endometrium 3 to 5 days
    before normal menses

Test explanation

An endometrial biopsy can determine whether ovulation has occurred. A biopsy specimen taken 3 to 5 days before normal menses should demonstrate a "secretory-type" endometrium on histologic examination if ovulation and corpus luteum formation have occurred. If not, only a preovulatory "proliferative-type" endometrium will be seen.

Another major use of endometrial biopsy is to diagnose endometrial cancer, tuberculosis, polyps, or inflammatory conditions or to evaluate uterine bleeding.

Potential complications

- Perforation of the uterus
- Uterine bleeding
- Interference with early pregnancy
- Infection

Procedure and patient care

Before

- Ensure that written and informed consent for this procedure is obtained from the patient.
- Tell the patient that no fasting or sedation is usually required.

During

- Note the following procedural steps:
    1. The cervix is exposed and cleansed.
    2. A biopsy instrument is inserted into the uterus, and specimens are obtained from the anterior, posterior, and lateral walls. This can be performed as a part of a D&C or hysteroscopy.
    3. The specimens are placed in a solution containing 10% formalin.

- Note that this procedure is performed by an obstetrician/gynecologist in approximately 10 to 30 minutes.

After

- Advise the patient to wear a pad because some vaginal bleeding is to be expected. Instruct the patient to call her physician if excessive bleeding (requiring more than one pad per hour) occurs.
- Inform the patient that douching and intercourse are not permitted for 72 hours after biopsy specimen removal.
- Instruct the patient to rest during the next 24 hours and to avoid heavy lifting to prevent uterine hemorrhage.

Abnormal findings

Anovulation
Tumor
Tuberculosis
Polyps
Inflammatory condition

notes

Epstein-Barr virus titer (EBV)

Type of test Blood

Normal findings

Titers ≤1:10 are nondiagnostic.

Titers of 1:10 to 1:60 indicate infection at some undetermined time.

Titers of 1:320 or greater suggest active infection.

Fourfold increase in titer in paired sera drawn 10 to 14 days apart is usually indicative of an acute infection.

Test explanation

In Africa EBV has been associated with Burkitt's lymphoma. In China EBV infection has been associated with nasopharyngeal carcinoma. In the United States, EBV titer is usually used to detect mononucleosis and other EBV infections.

Serologic tests are the only way to make a diagnosis of EBV. The heterophil agglutination slide test (monospot test) is one of the oldest tests used. Other, more specific immunologic tests indicate more precisely the timing of the infection. The viral capsid antigen-antibodies (VCAs) can be IgG or IgM. The EBV nuclear antigen (EBNA) is located in the nuclei of the infected lymphocyte. Early antigens (EA) have also been identified and assist in the diagnosis of EBV infections.

The interpretation of EBV antibody tests is based on the following assumptions:

1. Once the person becomes infected with EBV, the antiVCA antibodies appear first.
2. Anti-EA (EA-D or EA-R) antibodies appear next or are present with anti-VCA antibodies early in the course of illness. An anti-EA antibody titer greater than 80 in a patient 2 years after acute infectious mononucleosis indicates chronic EBV syndrome.
3. As the patient recovers, anti-VCA and anti-EA antibodies decrease, and anti-EBNA antibodies appear. Anti-EBNA antibody persists for life and reflects a past infection.
4. After the patient is well, anti-VCA and anti-EBNA antibodies are always present but at lower ranges. Occasionally anti-EA antibody also may be present after the patient recovers.

Procedure and patient care

Before

- Tell the patient that no fasting or special preparation is required.

During

- Collect 5 to 10 ml of venous blood in a red-top tube.
- Record the day of onset of illness on the laboratory slip.
- Obtain serum samples as soon as possible after the onset of the illness.
- Obtain a second blood specimen 14 to 21 days later.

After

- Apply pressure to the venipuncture site.

Abnormal findings

Infectious mononucleosis
Chronic fatigue syndrome
Chronic EBV carrier state
Burkitt's lymphoma
Nasopharyngeal cancer

notes

erythrocyte sedimentation rate (ESR, Sed rate test)

Type of test Blood

Normal findings

Westergren method
Male: up to 15 mm/hr
Female: up to 20 mm/hr
Child: up to 10 mm/hr
Newborn: 0-2 mm/hr

Test explanation

ESR is a measurement of the rate with which the red blood cells (RBCs) settle in saline or plasma over a specified time period. It is nonspecific and therefore not diagnostic for any particular organ disease or injury. Because acute and chronic infection, inflammation (collagen-vascular diseases), advanced neoplasm, and tissue necrosis or infarction increase the protein (mainly fibrinogen) content of plasma, RBCs have a tendency to stack up on one another, increasing their weight and causing them to descend faster. Therefore in these diseases the ESR is increased.

The ESR is a fairly reliable indicator of the course of disease and therefore can be used to monitor disease therapy, especially for inflammatory autoimmune diseases such as temporal arteritis or polymyalgia rheumatica. In general, as the disease worsens, the ESR increases; as the disease improves, the ESR decreases.

Interfering factors

- Artificially low results can occur when the collected specimen is allowed to stand longer than 3 hours before the testing.
- Pregnancy (second and third trimester) can cause elevated levels.

Procedure and patient care

Before
- Hold medications that may affect test results if indicated.

During
- Collect approximately 5 to 10 ml of venous blood in a lavender-top tube.

After
- Apply pressure to the venipuncture site.
- Transport the specimen immediately to the laboratory.

Abnormal findings

▲ **Increased levels**
Chronic renal failure
Malignant diseases
Bacterial infection
Inflammatory diseases
Necrotic tissue diseases
Hyperfibrinogenemia
Macroglobulinemia
Severe anemias such as iron
deficiency or B_{12} deficiency

▼ **Decreased levels**
Sickle cell anemia
Spherocytosis
Hypofibrinogenemia
Polycythemia vera

notes

ethanol (Ethyl alcohol, Blood alcohol, Blood EtOH)

Type of test Blood; urine; gastric; breath

Normal findings None

Possible critical values >300 mg/dl

Test explanation

This test is usually performed to evaluate alcohol-impaired driving or overdose. Proper collection, handling, and storage of blood alcohol are important for medicolegal cases involving sobriety. The blood test is the specimen of choice. Blood is taken from a peripheral vein in living patients and from the aorta in cadavers. Ethanol also can be detected in the urine, in gastric contents, or by breath analyzer. Blood alcohol levels between 50 to 100 mg/dl (0.05% to 0.10% weight/volume) are considered legal intoxication.

Interfering factors

- Elevated blood ketones (as with diabetic ketoacidosis) can cause false elevation of blood and breath test results.

Procedure and patient care

Before
- Follow the institution's protocol if the specimen will be used for legal purposes.

During
- Use a povidone-iodine wipe instead of an alcohol wipe for cleansing the venipuncture site.
- Collect a venous blood sample in a gray- or red-top tube according to the agency's protocol.
- If a gastric or urine specimen is indicated, approximately 20 to 50 ml of fluid is necessary.
- Breath analyzers are taken at the end of expiration after a deep inspiration.

After
- Apply pressure to the venipuncture site.
- Follow the agency's protocol regarding specimen collection.
- The exact time of specimen collection should be indicated. Also, in some instances signatures of the collector and a witness may be needed for legal evidence.

Abnormal findings

Alcohol intoxication or overdose

notes

fetal contraction stress test (CST, Oxytocin challenge test [OCT])

Type of test Electrodiagnostic

Normal findings Negative

Test explanation

CST, frequently called the *oxytocin challenge test* (OCT), is a relatively noninvasive test of fetoplacental adequacy used in the assessment of high-risk pregnancy. For this study a temporary stress in the form of uterine contractions is applied to the fetus after the IV administration of oxytocin. The reaction of the fetus to the contractions is assessed by an external fetal heart monitor. Uterine contractions cause transient impediment of placental blood flow. If the placental reserve is adequate, the maternal-fetal oxygen transfer is not significantly compromised during the contractions, and the fetal heart rate (FHR) remains normal (a *negative* test). The fetoplacental unit can then be considered adequate for the next 7 days.

If the placental reserve is inadequate, the fetus does not receive enough oxygen during the contraction. This results in intrauterine hypoxia and late deceleration of the FHR. The test is considered to be *positive* if consistent, persistent, late decelerations of the FHR occur with two or more uterine contractions.

Contraindications

- Patient pregnant with multiple fetuses because the myometrium is under greater tension and is more likely to be stimulated to premature labor
- Patient with a prematurely ruptured membrane because labor may be stimulated by the CST
- Patient with placenta previa because vaginal delivery may be induced
- Patient with abruptio placentae because the placenta may separate from the uterus as a result of the oxytocin-induced uterine contractions
- Patient with a previous hysterotomy because the strong uterine contractions may cause uterine rupture

Potential complications

- Premature labor

Procedure and patient care

Before
- Obtain informed consent for the procedure.
- Teach the patient breathing and relaxation techniques.
- Record the patient's blood pressure and FHR before the test as baseline values.
- If the CST is performed on an elective basis, the patient may be kept NPO in case labor occurs.

F

During
- Note the following procedural steps:
  1. Check the patient's blood pressure every 10 minutes to identify hypotension, which may cause diminished placental blood flow and a false-positive test result.
  2. Place an external fetal monitor and tocodynameter over the patient's abdomen to record the fetal heart tones and uterine contractions.
  3. Monitor baseline FHR and uterine activity for 20 minutes.
  4. If uterine contractions are detected during this pretest period, withhold oxytocin and monitor the response of the fetal heart tone to spontaneous uterine contractions.
  5. If no spontaneous uterine contractions occur, administer oxytocin (Pitocin) by IV infusion pump.
  6. Increase the rate of oxytocin infusion until the patient is having moderate contractions; then record the FHR pattern.
  7. After the oxytocin infusion is discontinued, continue FHR monitoring for another 30 minutes until the uterine activity has returned to its preoxytocin state. The body metabolizes oxytocin in approximately 20 to 25 minutes.
- Note that the CST is performed safely on an outpatient basis in the labor and delivery unit, where qualified nurses and necessary equipment are available.
- Note that the duration of this study is approximately 2 hours.
- Tell the patient that the discomfort associated with the CST may consist of mild labor contractions. Usually, breathing exercises are sufficient to control any discomfort. Administer analgesics if needed.

After
- Monitor the patient's blood pressure and the FHR.
- Discontinue the IV line and assess the site for bleeding.

Abnormal finding

Fetoplacental inadequacy

notes

fetal nonstress test (Nonstress test [NST], Fetal activity determination)

Type of test   Electrodiagnostic

Normal findings   "Reactive" fetus (heart rate acceleration associated with fetal movement)

F

Test explanation

NST is a method of evaluating the viability of a fetus. It documents the function of the placenta in its ability to supply adequate blood to the fetus. The NST can be used to evaluate any high-risk pregnancy in which fetal well-being may be threatened.

The NST is a noninvasive study that monitors acceleration of the fetal heart rate (FHR) in response to fetal movement. This FHR acceleration reflects the integrity of the central nervous system and fetal well-being. Fetal response is characterized as "reactive" or "nonreactive." The NST indicates a *reactive fetus* when, with fetal movement, two or more FHR accelerations are detected, each of which must be at least 15 beats/min for 15 seconds or more within any 10-minute period. The test is 99% reliable in indicating fetal well-being.

Procedure and patient care

Before

- If the patient is hungry, instruct her to eat before the NST is begun. Fetal activity is enhanced with a high maternal serum glucose level.

During

- Place an external fetal monitor on the patient's abdomen to record the FHR. The mother can indicate fetal movement by pressing a button on the fetal monitor whenever she feels the fetus move. FHR and fetal movement are concomitantly recorded on a two-channel strip graph.
- Observe the fetal monitor for FHR accelerations associated with fetal movement.
- If the fetus is quiet for 20 minutes, stimulate fetal activity by external methods such as rubbing or compressing the mother's abdomen, ringing a bell near the abdomen, or placing a pan on the abdomen and hitting the pan.

After

- If the results detect a nonreactive fetus, inform the patient that she is a candidate for the CST.

Abnormal findings

Fetal stress
Fetal death

notes

gallbladder nuclear scanning (Hepatobiliary scintigraphy, Hepatobiliary imaging, Biliary tract radionuclide scan, Cholescintigraphy, DISIDA scanning, HIDA scanning, IDA gallbladder scanning)

Type of test Nuclear scan

Normal findings Gallbladder, common bile duct, and duodenum visualized within 60 minutes after radionuclide injection. (This confirms patency of the cystic and common bile ducts.)

G

Test explanation

Through the use of iminodiacetic acid analogs (IDAs) labeled with technetium-99m (^{99m}Tc), the biliary tract can be evaluated in a safe, accurate, and noninvasive manner.

Failure to visualize the gallbladder 60 to 120 minutes after injection of the radionuclide dye is virtually diagnostic of an obstruction of the cystic duct (acute cholecystitis). Delayed filling of the gallbladder is associated with chronic or acalculus cholecystitis. The identification of the radionuclide in the biliary tree, but not in the bowel, is diagnostic of common bile duct obstruction.

With *cholescintigraphy*, gallbladder function can be numerically determined by calculating the capability of the gallbladder to eject its contents. It is believed that an ejection fraction below 35% indicates chronic cholecystitis or functional obstruction of the cystic duct.

Contraindications

- Pregnancy because of the risk of fetal damage

Interfering factors

- If the patient has not eaten for more than 24 hours, the radionuclide may not fill the gallbladder. This would produce a false-positive result.

Procedure and patient care

Before
- Instruct the patient to fast for at least 2 hours before the test. This fasting is preferable but not mandatory.

During

- Note the following procedural steps:
  1. After IV administration of a ^{99m}Tc-labeled IDA analog (e.g., DISIDA, PIPIDA, HIDA), the right upper quadrant of the abdomen is scanned.
  2. If the gallbladder, common bile duct, or duodenum are not visualized within 60 minutes after injection, delayed images are obtained up to 4 hours later.

After

- Obtain a meal for the patient if indicated.

Abnormal findings

Acute cholecystitis
Chronic cholecystitis
Acalculus cholecystitis
Common bile duct obstruction secondary to gallstones, tumor, or stricture
Cystic duct syndrome

notes

gamma-glutamyl transpeptidase (GGTP, γ-GTP, Gamma-glutamyl transferase [GGT])

Type of test Blood

Normal findings

Male and female over age 45: 8-38 U/L
Female under age 45: 5-27 U/L
Elderly: slightly higher than adult level
Child: similar to adult level
Newborn: 5 times higher than adult level

Test explanation

Highest concentrations of GGTP enzyme are found in the liver and biliary tract. Lesser concentration are found in the kidney, spleen, heart, intestine, brain, and prostate gland. This test is used to detect liver cell dysfunction, and it very accurately indicates even the slightest degree of cholestasis. This is the most sensitive liver enzyme in detecting biliary obstruction, cholangitis, or cholecystitis.

Another important clinical aspect of GGTP is that it can detect chronic alcohol ingestion. Therefore it is very useful in the screening and evaluation of alcoholic patients. GGTP is elevated in approximately 75% of patients who chronically drink alcohol.

Interfering factors

- Values may be decreased in late pregnancy.
- Drugs that may cause *increased* GGTP levels include alcohol, phenytoin (Dilantin), and phenobarbital.

Procedure and patient care

Before
- Tell the patient that an 8-hour fast is recommended. Only water is permitted.

During
- Collect approximately 7 to 10 ml of venous blood in a red-top tube.

After
- Apply pressure to the venipuncture site. Patients with liver dysfunction often have prolonged clotting times.

Abnormal findings

▲ **Increased levels**
  Hepatitis
  Cirrhosis
  Hepatic necrosis
  Hepatic tumor or metastasis
  Hepatotoxic drugs
  Cholestasis
  Jaundice
  Myocardial infarction
  Alcohol ingestion
  Pancreatitis
  Cancer of the pancreas
  Epstein Barr (infectious mononucleosis)
  Cytomegalovirus infections
  Reye's syndrome

notes

GASTROINTESTINAL ENDOSCOPY

esophagogastroduodenoscopy (EGD, Upper gastrointestinal [UGI] endoscopy, Gastroscopy)
endoscopic retrograde cholangiopancreatography (ERCP, ERCP of the biliary and pancreatic ducts)
colonoscopy
sigmoidoscopy (Proctoscopy, Anoscopy)

G

Type of test Endoscopy

Normal findings

Normal esophagus, stomach, and duodenum
Normal size of biliary and pancreatic ducts
No obstruction or filling defects within the biliary or pancreatic ducts
Normal colon

Test explanation

Endoscopy enables direct visualization of the gastrointestinal (GI) tract by means of a long, flexible, fiberoptic-lighted scope. The esophagus, stomach, duodenum, colon, and rectum are examined for tumors, varices, mucosal inflammations, hiatal hernias, polyps, ulcers, and obstructions. Through the scope, pathology can be visualized and biopsied. Probes can also be passed to allow for coagulation or injection of sclerosing agents to areas of active GI bleeding. A laser beam can pass through the endoscope to perform endoscopic surgery (e.g., obliteration of tumors or polyps, control of bleeding), and the fiberoptics of endoscopy are so refined that video images and "still pictures" can be taken.

EGD is used to evaluate patients with dysphagia, weight loss, early satiety, upper abdominal pain, "ulcer symptoms," or dyspepsia. It is also used to detect esophageal varices in alcoholics. Suspicious barium swallow or upper GI x-ray findings can be corroborated by EGD. With endoscopy, one can not only evaluate the esophagus, stomach, and duodenum, but, with the use of an extralong fiberoptic endoscope, one can also visualize and perform a biopsy of tissue in the upper small intestinal tract.

With the use of a fiberoptic endoscope, ERCP provides radiographic visualization of the bile and pancreatic ducts. This is especially useful in patients with jaundice. If a partial or total obstruction of those ducts exists, characteristics of the obstructing lesion can be demonstrated. Stones, benign strictures, cysts, ampullary stenosis, anatomic variations, and malignant tumors can be identified. Stents can be placed through strictured bile ducts with the use of ERCP, and the bile of jaundiced patients can be internally drained.

With fiberoptic colonoscopy, the entire colon from anus to cecum can be examined in most patients. Shorter scopes are used to examine the more distal parts of the colon. *Anoscopy* refers to examination of the anus, *proctoscopy* to examination of the anus and rectum, and *sigmoidoscopy* (the most frequent procedure) to examination of the anus, rectum, and sigmoid colon. Colonoscopy is recommended for patients who have obvious or occult blood in the stools, lower gastrointestinal bleeding, or a change in bowel habits or are at high risk for colon cancer. It is also recommended for patients who have abdominal pain and is used as a surveillance tool for patients who have had colorectal cancer, inflammatory bowel disease, or polyposis.

Furthermore, sigmoidoscopy, as with colonoscopy, can be therapeutic. Reduction of sigmoid volvulus, removal of polyps, and obliteration of hemorrhoids can be performed through the sigmoidoscope.

Contraindications

- Patients who cannot cooperate fully
- Patients with severe GI bleeding
- Patients with esophageal diverticula
- Patients with suspected perforation
- Patients who have had recent GI surgery
- Patients whose ampulla of Vater is not accessible endoscopically because of previous upper gastrointestinal surgery

Potential complications

- Perforation of the gut
- Bleeding from a biopsy site
- Oversedation from the medication administered during the test
- Pancreatitis, which can be induced with injection of dye into the pancreatic duct

Interfering factors

- Food in the stomach
- Excessive GI bleeding

- Barium in the GI tract, which may preclude visualization of the pancreatic-biliary tree
- Stool immediately obstructing the lens and precluding adequate visualization of the colon

Procedure and patient care

Before

- Explain the procedure to the patient.
- Obtain informed consent if required by the institution.
- Instruct the patient to abstain from eating as of midnight the day of the test.
- Instruct the patient not to bite down on the endoscope for EGD.
- For lower GI endoscopy:
  1. A *1-day preparation* using a glycol (COLyte) bowel preparation has become widely used. The 1 gallon should be consumed within 4 hours if possible on the day prior to the test.
  2. Administer appropriate preendoscopy sedation, usually meperidine (Demerol) and diazepam (Valium). Often atropine is ordered to minimize patient secretions.

During

- For upper GI endoscopy:
  1. The patient is placed on the endoscopy table in the left lateral decubitus position.
  2. The throat is topically anesthetized with viscous lidocaine (Xylocaine) or another anesthetic spray.
  3. The patient is sedated.
  4. The endoscope is gently passed through the mouth and finally into the esophagus; once in the esophagus, visualization can be performed.
  5. Air is insufflated to distend the upper GI tract for adequate visualization.
  6. The esophagus, stomach, and duodenum are evaluated.
- For ERCP:
  1. A flat plate of the abdomen is taken to ensure that any barium from previous studies will not obscure visualization of the bile duct.
  2. The procedure is the same as EGD except that a side-viewing fiberoptic duodenoscope is inserted and passed through the esophagus and stomach and into the duodenum.

G

3. Through the accessory lumen within the scope, a small catheter is passed through the ampulla and into the common bile or pancreatic ducts.
4. Radiographic dye is injected, and x-ray films are taken.

- For lower GI endoscopy:
  1. After a rectal examination indicates adequate bowel preparation, the patient is sedated (not required for sigmoidoscopy).
  2. The patient is placed in the lateral decubitus position, and the colonoscope or sigmoidoscope is placed into the rectum.
  3. Under direct visualization, the colonoscope is directed to the cecum. Often a significant amount of manipulation is required to obtain this position.
  4. As in all endoscopy, air is insufflated to distend the bowel for better visualization.

After

- Inform the patient that he or she may have hoarseness or a sore throat after EGD or ERCP.
- Withhold any fluids until the patient is completely alert and the swallowing reflex returns to normal, usually 2 to 4 hours.
- Observe the patient's vital signs. Evaluate the patient for bleeding, fever, abdominal pain, dyspnea, or dysphagia.
- Inform the patient that he or she may experience some post-endoscopic bloating, belching, and flatulence.
- Inform the patient that the sedation may cause some retrograde and antegrade amnesia for a few hours.
- If a bowel preparation was used, encourage the patient to drink fluids after the test.

Abnormal findings

Tumor (benign or malignant) of the esophagus, stomach, or duodenum

Esophageal diverticula

Hiatal hernia

Esophagitis, gastritis, duodenitis

Gastroesophageal varices

Peptic ulcer

Peptic stricture and subsequent scarring

Extrinsic compression by a cyst or tumor outside the upper GI tract

Upper GI bleeding

Tumor, strictures, or gallstones of the common bile duct

Sclerosing cholangitis

Biliary sclerosis

Cysts of the common bile duct

Tumor, strictures, or inflammation of the pancreatic duct

Pseudocyst of the pancreatic duct

Chronic pancreatitis

Anatomic biliary or pancreatic duct variations

Cancer of the duodenum or ampulla

Colorectal cancer

Colorectal polyps

Inflammatory bowel disease (e.g., ulcerative or Crohn's colitis)

AV malformations

Hemorrhoids

Ischemic or postinflammatory strictures

Diverticulosis

G

notes

GLUCOSE STUDIES

glucose, blood (Blood sugar, Fasting blood sugar [FBS])
glucose, urine (Urine sugar)

Type of test Blood, urine

Normal findings

Blood:
 Neonate: 30-60 mg/dl or 1.7-3.3 mmol/L
 Infant: 40-90 mg/dl or 2.2-5.0 mmol/L
 Child <2 years: 60-100 mg/dl or 3.3-5.5 mmol/L
 Child >2 years to adult: 70-105 mg/dl or 3.9-5.8 mmol/L
 Elderly: increase in normal range after age 50 years
Urine:
 Random specimen: No glucose noted
 24-hour specimen: <0.5 g/day or <2.78 mmol/day (SI units)

Possible critical values

Blood:
 Adult male: <50 and >400 mg/dl
 Adult female: <40 and >400 mg/dl
 Infant: <40 mg/dl

Test explanation

Through an elaborate feedback mechanism, glucose levels are controlled by insulin and glucagon. In general, true glucose elevations indicate diabetes mellitus; however, there are many other possible causes of hyperglycemia. Similarly, hypoglycemia has many causes. The most common cause is inadvertent insulin overdose in patients with brittle diabetes.

Serum glucose levels must be evaluated according to the time of day they are performed. For example, a glucose level of 135 mg/dl may be abnormal if the patient is in the fasting state, but this level would be within normal limits if the patient had eaten a meal within the last hour.

Glucose determinations must be performed frequently in new patients with diabetes to monitor closely the insulin dosage to be administered. Finger stick blood glucose determinations are often performed before meals and at bedtime. Results are compared with a sliding-scale insulin chart ordered by the physician to provide coverage with SQ regular insulin.

A glucose test is usually part of a routine urinalysis. This screening test for the presence of glucose within the urine may indicate the likelihood of diabetes mellitus or other causes of glucose intolerance. Urine glucose tests are also used to monitor the effectiveness of diabetes therapy; however, this is largely supplanted today by finger stick determinations of blood glucose levels.

Glucose is filtered from the blood by the glomeruli of the kidney. Normally, all of the glucose is resorbed in the proximal renal tubules. When the blood glucose level exceeds the capability of the renal threshold to resorb the glucose (normally, around 180 mg/dl), it begins to spill over into the urine (glycosuria). As the blood glucose level increases further, greater amounts of glucose are spilled into the urine. In patients who do not have diabetes, glucosuria can occur with a normal serum glucose level when kidney diseases affect the renal tubule. The renal threshold for glucose becomes abnormally low, and glucosuria occurs.

Interfering factors

- Physical stress can cause increased serum glucose levels.
- Most patients receiving dextrose-containing IV fluids will have increased glucose levels.
- Many pregnant women experience some degree of glucose intolerance. If significant, it is called gestational diabetes.
- Drugs that may cause *increased* glucose levels include corticosteroids, diuretics, epinephrine, and glucagon, among others.
- Drugs that may cause *decreased* glucose levels include alcohol, insulin, monoamine oxidase inhibitors, pentamidine, and oral hypoglycemic agents.
- Any substance that can reduce the copper in Clinitest can produce positive urine results. This may include other sugars such as galactose, fructose, or lactose.

Procedure and patient care

Before

- For FBS, keep the patient fasting at least 8 hours. Water is permitted.
- Withhold insulin or oral hypoglycemics until after blood is obtained.

During

- Blood:
  1. Collect approximately 7 ml of venous blood in a red- or gray-top tube.
  2. Glucose levels can also be evaluated by performing a finger stick and using either a visually read strip or a reflectance meter (e.g., Glucometer, Accu Check, Stat Tek).
- Urine:
  3. Because accuracy is necessary, collect a "fresh" urine specimen. The stagnant urine that has been in the bladder for several hours will not accurately reflect the serum glucose level at testing.
  4. Collect a urine specimen 30 to 40 minutes before the time the urine specimen is actually needed.
  5. Obtain a *double-voided specimen* and discard the first specimen.
  6. At the required time, obtain a second specimen, which is tested for glucose.
  7. Inform the patient that testing for glucose can be performed easily using enzyme tests such as Clinistix, Diastix, or Tes-Tape.

After

- Be certain that the patient receives a meal after fasting blood work.

Abnormal findings

▲ **Increased levels
   (hyperglycemia)**
   Blood
   Diabetes mellitus
   Acute stress response
   Cushing's syndrome
   Pheochromocytoma
   Chronic renal failure
   Glucagonoma
   Acute pancreatitis
   Diuretic therapy
   Corticosteroid therapy
   Acromegaly
   Urine
   Diabetes mellitus
   Acute stress response
   Cushing's syndrome
   Pheochromocytoma
   Pregnancy
   Renal glycosuria
   Hereditary defects in
     metabolism of other
     reducing substance
     (e.g., galactose, fruc-
     tose, pentose)
   Nephrotoxic chemicals
     (e.g., carbon monoxide,
     mercury, lead)

▼ **Decreased levels
   (hypoglycemia)**
   Insulinoma
   Hypothyroidism
   Hypopituitarism
   Addison's disease
   Extensive liver disease
   Insulin overdose
   Starvation

G

notes

glucose tolerance test and postprandial glucose (GTT, Oral glucose tolerance test [OGTT], 2-hour postprandial glucose [2-hour PPG], 2-hour postprandial blood sugar, 1-hour glucose screen for gestational diabetes mellitus)

Type of test   Blood; urine

Normal findings

Serum test

Fasting: 70-115 mg/dl or <6.4 mmol/L (SI units)
30 minutes: <200 mg/dl or <11.1 mmol/L
1 hour: <200 mg/dl or <11.1 mmol/L
2 hours: <140 mg/dl or <7.8 mmol/L
3 hours: 70-115 mg/dl or <6.4 mmol/L
4 hours: 70-115 mg/dl or <6.4 mmol/L

1-hour glucose screen for gestational diabetes
<140 mg/dl

Urine test
Negative

Test explanation

A GTT peak and 2-hour value of greater than 200 mg/100 ml on more than one occasion is one of the National Diabetes Data Group (NDDG)'s criteria for the diagnosis of DM. The GTT is used when diabetes is suspected (retinopathy, neuropathy, diabetic-type renal diseases). It is also suggested for the following:

1. Patients with a family history of diabetes
2. Patients who are massively obese
3. Patients with a history of recurrent infections
4. Patients with delayed healing of wounds (especially on the lower legs or feet)
5. Women who have a history of delivering large babies or who have stillbirths
6. Patients who have transient glycosuria or hyperglycemia during pregnancy, following myocardial infarction, or following surgery or stress

In the GTT the patient's ability to tolerate a standard oral glucose load is evaluated by obtaining serum and urine specimens for glucose determinations before glucose administration and then at 30 minutes, 1 hour, 2 hours, 3 hours, and sometimes 4 hours afterwards. Patients with diabetes will not be able to tolerate this load. As a result, their serum glucose levels will be greatly elevated from 1 to 5 hours. Also, glucose can be detected in their urine.

The American Diabetes Association recommends that pregnant women who have not previously had an abnormal GTT should be tested at the 24th and 28th week of gestation with a 50-g dose of glucose. A glucose level of >140 mg/100 ml suggests that the women should be retested with a nonpregnant GTT 6 weeks or more after delivery.

Glucose intolerance also may exist in patients with oversecretion of hormones that have an ancillary affect on glucose, such as Cushing's syndrome, pheochromocytoma, acromegaly, aldosteronism, or hyperthyroidism. The GTT is also used to evaluate patients with reactive hypoglycemia. This may occur as late as 5 hours after the initial glucose load.

The postprandial glucose (PPG) test is an easily performed screening test for diabetes mellitus. If the results are >140 mg/dl and <200 mg/dl, a full glucose tolerance test may be performed to confirm the diagnosis. If the 2-hour PPG is >200 mg/dl, the diagnosis of diabetes mellitus is confirmed. For this study a meal acts as a glucose challenge to the body's metabolism. The *1-hour glucose screen* is used to detect gestational diabetes mellitus (GDM).

Contraindication

- Patients with serious concurrent infections or endocrine disorders because glucose intolerance will be observed even though these patients may not have diabetes

Potential complications

- Dizziness, tremors, anxiety, sweating, euphoria, or fainting during testing
- If these symptoms occur, a blood specimen is obtained. If the glucose level is too high, the test may need to be stopped and insulin administered.

Interfering factors

- Stress (e.g., from surgery, infection) can increase glucose levels.
- Exercise during the testing can affect glucose levels.
- Fasting or reduced caloric intake before GTT can cause glucose intolerance.

Procedure and patient care

Before

- For the *2-hour PPG*, instruct the patient to eat the entire meal (with at least 75 g of carbohydrates) and then not to eat anything else until the blood is drawn.
- For the *1-hour glucose screen for GDM*, give the fasting or nonfasting patient a 50-g oral glucose load.
- For the GTT:
  1. Educate the patient about the importance of having adequate food intake with adequate carbohydrates (150 g) for at least 3 days before the test.
  2. Instruct the patient to fast for 12 hours before the test.
  3. Obtain the patient's weight to determine the appropriate glucose loading dose (especially in children).

During

- Obtain fasting blood and urine specimens.
- Administer the oral glucose solution, usually a 75- to 100-g carbohydrate load.
- Give pediatric patients a carbohydrate load of 1.75 g/kg body weight, up to a maximum of 75 g.
- Instruct the patient to ingest the entire glucose load.
- Tell the patient that he or she cannot eat anything until the test is completed. However, encourage the patient to drink water. No other liquids should be taken.
- Collect approximately 5 ml of venous blood in a gray-top tube at 30 minutes and at hourly periods. Apply pressure or a pressure dressing to the sites.
- Collect urine specimens at hourly periods.
- For the IV-GTT, administer the glucose load intravenously over 3 to 4 minutes.

After

- Allow the patient to eat and drink normally.
- Administer insulin or oral hypoglycemics if ordered.

Abnormal findings

Diabetes mellitus	Chronic renal failure
Acute stress response	Glucagonoma
Cushing's syndrome	Acute pancreatitis
Pheochromocytoma	Acromegaly

glycosylated hemoglobin (GHb, GHB, Glycohemoglobin, Hemoglobin [Hb] A$_{1c}$, Diabetic control index)

Type of test Blood

Normal findings Vary with laboratory method used

Adult/elderly: 4% to 8%
Child: usually <7%
Good diabetic control: 7%
Fair diabetic control: 10%
Poor diabetic control: 13% to 20%

G

Test explanation

This test is used to monitor diabetes treatment. It measures the amount of glucose-laden hemoglobin A$_{1c}$ (HbA$_{1c}$) in the blood and provides an accurate long-term index of the patient's average blood glucose level.

The amount of glycosylated hemoglobin (glycohemoglobin [GHb]) depends on the amount of glucose available in the bloodstream over the RBCs' 120-day life span. Therefore determination of the GHb value reflects the average blood sugar level for the 100- to 120-day period before the test. One important advantage of this test is that the sample can be drawn at any time because it is not affected by short-term variations (e.g., food intake, exercise, stress, hypoglycemic agents, patient cooperation).

The GHb test is particularly beneficial for the following:

1. Evaluating the success and patient compliance of diabetic treatment
2. Comparing and contrasting the success of past and new forms of diabetic therapy
3. Determining the duration of hyperglycemia in patients with newly diagnosed diabetes
4. Providing a sensitive estimate of glucose imbalance in patients with mild diabetes
5. Individualizing diabetic control regimens
6. Providing a feeling of reward for many patients when the test shows achievement of good diabetic control
7. Evaluating the diabetic patient whose glucose levels change significantly day to day (brittle diabetic)
8. Differentiating short-term hyperglycemia in patients who do not have diabetes (e.g., recent stress or myocardial

infarction) from those who have diabetes (where the glucose has been persistently elevated).

Interfering factors

- Hemoglobinopathies can affect results because the quantity of hemoglobin A (and, as a result, HbA_1) varies considerably in these diseases.
- Falsely elevated values occur when the RBC life span is lengthened because the hemoglobin A_1 has a longer period available for glycosylation.

Procedure and patient care

Before
- Tell the patient that fasting is not indicated.

During
- Collect approximately 5 ml of venous blood in a gray- or lavender-top tube.

After
- Apply pressure to the venipuncture site.

Abnormal findings

▲ **Increased levels**
  Newly diagnosed diabetic patient
  Poorly controlled diabetic patient
  Nondiabetic hyperglycemia (e.g., acute stress response, Cushing's syndrome, pheochromocytoma, glucagonoma, corticosteroid therapy, or acromegaly)
  Splenectomized patients
  Pregnancy

▼ **Decreased levels**
  Hemolytic anemia
  Chronic blood loss
  Chronic renal failure

notes

Helicobacter pylori antibodies test

(*Campylobacter pylori*, Anti-*Helicobacter pylori* immunoglobulin G [IgG] antibody, Campylobacter-like organism [CLO] test)

Type of test   Blood, microscopic examination of antral or duodenal biopsy specimen, breath test

Normal findings   Not present

Test explanation

H

Helicobacter pylori infection has been incriminated as the cause of peptic ulcers and gastric cancer.

There are several methods of detecting the presence of *H. pylori*. It can be cultured from a specimen of mucus obtained through a gastroscope. The organism can also be detected on a gastric mucosal biopsy.

Immunoassays to serum antibodies to *H. pylori* have been developed and are very accurate in detecting the presence of the organism. The IgG anti-*H. pylori* antibody is most commonly used. It becomes elevated 2 months after infection and stays elevated for over a year after treatment. The IgA anti-*H. pylori* antibody, like IgG, becomes elevated 2 months after infection but decreases 3 to 4 weeks after treatment. The IgM anti-*H. pylori* antibody is the first to become elevated (about 3 to 4 weeks) and is not detected after 2 to 3 months after treatment. These antibody titers are fast becoming the "gold standard" for *H. pylori* detection.

There is also a *breath test* available for the detection of *H. pylori*. The breath test depends on the ability of *H. pylori* to break down urea into carbon dioxide and ammonia via its enzyme, urease. A dose of radioactive ^{14}C or nonradioactive ^{13}C urea is given by mouth. The isotopic CO_2 concentration is determined by breath collection.

Procedure and patient care

Before

- Tell the patient that no fasting is required for the blood test.
- If a biopsy or culture will be obtained by endoscopy, see discussion of esophagogastroduodenoscopy (EGD) (p. 137).

During

- Collect a venous blood sample according to the protocol of the laboratory performing the test.
- A gastric or duodenal biopsy can be obtained by endoscopy. Keep the specimen moist by the addition of approximately 5 ml of sterile saline.
- For the *breath test,* a dose of radioactive ^{14}C or nonradioactive ^{13}C urea is given by mouth.

After

- Apply pressure to the venipuncture site.
- If endoscopy was used to obtain a culture, see procedure for EGD (p. 137). The specimen should be transported to the laboratory within 30 minutes after collection.

Abnormal findings

▲   **Increased levels**
     Acute and chronic gastritis
     Duodenal ulcer
     Gastric ulcer
     Gastric carcinoma

notes

hemoglobin and hematocrit (Hb, Hgb, Hct, Packed red blood cell volume, Packed cell volume [PCV]) (H&H)

Type of tests Blood

Normal findings

Hemoglobin

Male: 14-18 g/dl or 8.7-11.2 mmol/L (SI units)
Female: 12-16 g/dl or 7.4-9.9 mmol/L
Pregnant female: >11 g/dl
Elderly: values are slightly decreased
Newborn: 14-24 g/dl
Children: 9.5-15 g/dl

Hematocrit

Male: 42%-52% or 0.42-0.52 volume fraction (SI units)
Female: 37%-47% or 0.37-0.47 volume fraction (SI units)
Pregnant female: >33%
Elderly: values may be slightly decreased
Newborn: 44-64
Children: 29-43

Possible critical values

Hemoglobin: <5.0 g/dl or >20 g/dl
Hematocrit: <15% or >60%

Test explanation

The Hgb concentration is a measure of the total amount of Hgb in the peripheral blood, which reflects the number of red blood cells (RBCs) in the blood. The Hct is a measure of the percentage of the total blood volume that is made up by the red blood cells (RBCs). The height of the RBC column is measured after centrifugation. It is compared to the height of the column of the total whole blood. The ratio of the height of the RBC column compared to the original total blood column is multiplied by 100%. This is the Hct value. These tests are normally performed as part of a *complete blood count (CBC)* or as a part of a H & H.

The hematocrit (Hct) in percentage points usually is approximately three times the Hgb concentration in grams/per deciliter when RBCs are of normal size and contain normal amounts of

Hgb. Abnormal values of hemoglobin and hematocrit (H&H) indicate the same pathologic states as abnormal RBC counts (see p. 241). Decreased levels indicate anemia (reduced number of RBCs). Increased levels can indicate erythrocytosis. Changes in plasma volume are reflected by the H&H. Overhydration decreases H&H, whereas dehydration increases H&H. Hemoglobinopathies such as sickle cell disease and Hgb C disease are also associated with reduced H&H levels.

Interfering factors

- Slight H&H decreases normally occur during pregnancy because of the expanded blood volume.
- Living in high-altitude areas causes high H&H values.
- Extremely elevated white blood cell counts may affect hematocrit values.

Procedure and patient care

Before

- Explain the procedure to the patient.
- Tell the patient that no fasting is required.

During

- Collect approximately 5 to 7 ml of venous blood in a lavender-top tube.
- Avoid hemolysis.

After

- Apply pressure to the venipuncture site.

Abnormal findings

▲ **Increased levels**
Congenital heart disease
Polycythemia vera
Hemoconcentration of the blood
Chronic obstructive pulmonary disease
Congestive heart failure
High altitudes
Severe burns
Dehydration

▼ **Decreased levels**
Anemia
Severe hemorrhage
Hemolysis
Hemoglobinopathies
Cancer
Nutritional deficiency
Systemic lupus erythematosus
Sarcoidosis
Kidney disease
Chronic hemorrhage
Splenomegaly
Sickle cell anemia

hemoglobin electrophoresis (Hgb electrophoresis)

Type of test Blood

Normal findings

Adult/elderly

Hgb A_1: 95% to 98%
Hgb A_2: 2% to 3%
Hgb F: 0.8% to 2%
Hgb S: 0%
Hgb C: 0%

Children: Hgb F

Newborn: 50% to 80%
6 months: 8%
>6 months: 1% to 2%

Test explanation

Hgb electrophoresis is a test that identifies abnormal forms of Hgb (hemoglobinopathies).

The form *Hgb A_1* constitutes the major component of Hgb in the normal red blood cell (RBC). *Hgb A_2* is only a minor component (2% to 3%) of the normal Hgb total. *Hgb F* is the major hemoglobin component in the fetus but normally exists in only minimal quantities in the normal adult. Levels of Hgb F greater than 2% in patients over 3 years of age are considered abnormal. Hgb F is able to transport oxygen when only small amounts of oxygen are available (as in fetal life). In patients requiring compensation for prolonged chronic hypoxia (as in congenital cardiac abnormalities), Hgb F may be found in increased levels to assist in the transport of the available oxygen.

Hgb S and *Hgb C* are abnormal forms of Hgb that occur predominantly in American blacks and cause sickle cell disease and Hemoglobin C disease, respectively.

Interfering factor

- Blood transfusions within the previous 12 weeks may alter test results.

Procedure and patient care

Before

- Tell the patient that no fasting is required.

During

- Collect approximately 7 ml of venous blood in a lavender-top tube.

After

- Apply pressure to the venipuncture site.

Abnormal findings

Sickle cell disease
Sickle cell trait
Hemoglobin C disease
Hemoglobin H disease
Thalassemia major
Thalassemia minor

notes

hepatitis virus studies (Hepatitis-associated antigen [HAA], Australian antigen)

Type of test Blood

Normal findings Negative

Test explanation

The three viruses now recognized as causing hepatitis are hepatitis A, hepatitis B, and hepatitis non-A/non-B (also called hepatitis C) viruses. Hepatitis D and E viruses are much less common in the United States. The various types of hepatitis cannot be differentiated on the basis of their clinical presentation.

Two types of antibodies to *hepatitis A virus (HAV)* can be detected. The first type of antibody to HAV is immunoglobulin (Ig) M antibody (HAV-Ab/IgM), which appears approximately 3 to 4 weeks after exposure and returns to normal in approximately 8 weeks.

The second type of antibody is IgG (HAV-Ab/IgG). The IgG antibody can remain detectable for more than 10 years after the infection. If the IgM antibody is elevated in the absence of the IgG antibody, acute hepatitis is suspected. If, however, IgG is elevated in the absence of IgM elevation, this indicates the convalescent or chronic stage of HAV viral infection.

Hepatitis B virus (HBV) also called the *Dane particle,* is made up of an inner core surrounded by an outer capsule. The outer capsule contains the hepatitis B surface antigen (HBsAg), formerly called Australian antigen. The inner core contains HBV core antigen (HBcAg). The hepatitis B e-antigen (HBeAg) is also found within the core. Antibodies to these antigens are called HBsAb, HBcAb, and HBeAb. The tests used to detect these antigens and antibodies include:

1. *Hepatitis B surface antigen (HBsAg).* This is the most frequently and easily performed test for hepatitis B, and this is the first test to become abnormal. HBsAg rises before the onset of clinical symptoms, peaks during the first week of symptoms, and returns to normal by the time jaundice subsides. HBsAg generally indicates active infection by HBV. If the level of this antigen persists in the blood, the patient is considered to be a carrier.

2. *Hepatitis B surface antibody (HBsAb).* This antibody appears approximately 4 weeks after the disappearance of

H

the surface antigen and signifies the end of the acute infection phase. HBsAb also signifies immunity to subsequent infection. Concentrated forms of this agent constitute the hyperimmunoglobulin given to patients who have come in contact with HBV-infected patients (e.g., contact by an inadvertent needle prick from a needle previously used on a patient with HBV infection). HBsAb is the antibody that denotes immunity after administration of hepatitis B vaccine.

3. *Hepatitis B core antigen (HBcAg)*. No tests are routinely available to detect this antigen.

4. *Hepatitis B core antibody (HBcAb)*. This antibody appears approximately 1 month after infection with HBsAg and declines (although it remains elevated) over several years. HBcAb is also present in patients with chronic hepatitis. The HBcAb level is elevated during the time lag between the disappearance of HBsAg and the appearance of HBsAb. This interval is called the "core window." During the core window, HBcAb is the only detectable marker of a recent hepatitis infection.

5. *Hepatitis B e-antigen (HBeAg)*. This antigen is generally not used for diagnostic purposes but rather as an index of infectivity. The presence of HBeAg correlates with early and active disease, as well as with high infectivity in acute HBV infection. The persistent presence of HBeAg in the blood predicts the development of chronic HBV infection.

6. *Hepatitis B e-antibody (HBeAb)*. This antibody indicates that an acute phase of HBV infection is over, or almost over, and that the chance of infectivity is greatly reduced.

Non-A, non-B hepatitis (NANB), also called *hepatitis C (HCV)*, is transmitted in a manner similar to that of HBV. The incubation period is 2 to 12 weeks after exposure. An HCV viral titer to detect HCV IgG antibodies is now available to detect these infections; however, no vaccine protection exists against this form of hepatitis.

Hepatitis D virus (HDV) is known to cause "delta hepatitis." The HDV antigen can be detected by immunoassay within a few days after infection. The IgM and total antibodies to HDV are detected early in the disease also. A persistent elevation of these antibodies indicates a chronic or carrier state.

Hepatitis E virus (HEV) was initially included in the NANB virus group but was isolated several years ago. No antigen or an-

tibody tests are currently widely available or accurate for serologic testing.

Procedure and patient care

Before
- Tell the patient that no fasting is required.

During
- Collect approximately 5 to 7 ml of venous blood in a red-
top tube.
- Note that most of the testing for hepatitis is done by radio-
immunoassay. Usually a hepatitis profile that includes several
HBV antigens and antibodies is performed.

After
- Apply pressure to the venipuncture site.
- Handle the specimen as if it were capable of transmitting
hepatitis.

Abnormal findings

▲ **Increased levels**
Hepatitis A
Hepatitis B
Non-A, non-B hepatitis
Chronic carrier state, hepatitis B
Chronic hepatitis B

notes

holter monitoring (Ambulatory monitoring, Ambulatory electrocardiography, Event recorder)

Type of test Electrodiagnostic

Normal findings Normal sinus rhythm

Test explanation

Holter monitoring is a continuous recording of the electrical activity of the heart. With this technique an electrocardiogram (ECG) is recorded continuously on magnetic tape during unrestricted activity, rest, and sleep. The Holter monitor is equipped with a clock that permits accurate time monitoring on the ECG tape. The patient is asked to carry a diary and record daily activities, as well as any cardiac symptoms that may develop during the period of monitoring.

The Holter monitor is used primarily to identify suspected cardiac rhythm disturbances and to correlate these disturbances with symptoms such as dizziness, syncope, palpitations, or chest pain. The monitor is also used to assess pacemaker function and the effectiveness of antiarrhythmic medications.

After completion of the determined time period, usually 24 to 72 hours, the Holter monitor is removed from the patient, and the record tape is played back at high speeds. The ECG tracing is usually interpreted by computer, which can detect any significant abnormal waveform patterns that occurred during the testing.

Contraindications

- Patients who are unable to cooperate with maintaining the lead placement from the monitor to the body

Interfering factor

- Interruption in the electrode contact with the skin

Procedure and patient care

Before

- Inform the patient about the necessity of ensuring good contact between the electrodes and the skin.
- Teach the patient how to maintain an accurate diary. Stress the need to record significant symptoms.
- Instruct the patient not to bathe during the period of cardiac monitoring.

- Tell the patient to minimize the use of electrical devices (e.g., electric toothbrushes, shavers), which may cause artificial changes in the ECG tracing.

During

- Place the gel and electrodes at the appropriate sites. Usually the chest and abdomen are the most appropriate locations for limb-lead electrode placement. The precordial leads also may be placed.
- Encourage the patient to call if he or she has any difficulties.

After

- Gently remove the tape and other paraphernalia securing the electrodes.
- Wipe the patient clean of electrode gel.
- Inform the patient that the Holter monitoring interpretation will be available in a few days.

Abnormal findings

Cardiac arrhythmia (dysrhythmia)
Ischemic changes

notes

immunoglobulin electrophoresis (Gamma globulin electrophoresis)

Type of test Blood

Normal findings

IgG (mg/dl)
  Adults: 565-1765
  Children: 250-1600
IgA (mg/dl)
  Adults: 85-385
  Children: 1-350
IgM (mg/dl)
  Adult: 55-375
  Children: 20-200
IgD and IgE: minimal

Test explanation

  Serum immunoelectrophoresis is used to detect and monitor the course of diseases, including hypersensitivity diseases, immune deficiencies, autoimmune diseases, chronic infections, multiple myeloma, chronic viral infections, and intrauterine fetal infections. Immunoglobulins are separated out and electrophoresed according to the quantity and difference in electrical charge. Specific antisera are placed alongside the slide to identify the specific type of immunoglobulin present.

Procedure and patient care

Before
- Tell the patient that no fasting or special preparation is required.

During
- Collect 7 to 10 ml of venous blood in a red-top tube.
- Indicate on the laboratory slip if the patient has received any vaccinations or immunizations within the past 6 months. Also, list any drugs that may affect test results.

After
- Apply pressure to the venipuncture site.

Abnormal findings

▲ **Increased IgA levels**
Chronic liver diseases
(e.g., primary biliary
cirrhosis)
Chronic infections
Inflammatory bowel
disease

▼ **Decreased IgA levels**
Ataxia/telangiectasia
Congenital isolated defi-
ciency
Hypoproteinemia (e.g.,
nephrotic syndrome or
protein-losing enteropa-
thies)
Immunosuppressive
drugs (e.g., steroids,
dextran)

▲ **Increased IgG levels**
Chronic granulomatous
infections (e.g., tuber-
culosis, Wegener's
granulomatosis, sarcoid-
osis)
Hyper-immunization re-
actions
Chronic liver disease
Multiple myeloma
(monoclonal IgG type)
Autoimmune diseases
(e.g., rheumatoid ar-
thritis, Sjögren's
disease, and SLE)
IUD devices

▼ **Decreased IgG levels**
Wiskott-Aldrich syn-
drome
Agammaglobulinemia
AIDS
Hypoproteinemia (e.g.,
nephrotic syndrome or
protein-losing enteropa-
thies)
Drug immunosuppres-
sion (e.g., steroids,
dextran)
Non-IgG multiple
myeloma
Leukemia

▲ **Increased IgM levels**
Waldenström's macro-
globulinemia
Chronic infections (e.g.,
hepatitis, mononucleo-
sis, sarcoidosis)
Autoimmune diseases
(e.g., SLE or rheuma-
toid arthritis)
Acute infections
Chronic liver disorders
(e.g., biliary cirrhosis)

▼ **Decreased IgM levels**
Agammaglobulinemia
AIDS
Hypoproteinemia (e.g.,
nephrotic syndrome or
protein-losing enteropa-
thies)
Drug immunosuppres-
sion (e.g., steroids,
dextran)
IgG or IgA multiple
myeloma
Leukemia

▲ **Increased IgE levels**
Allergy reactions (e.g.,
   hayfever, asthma,
   eczema, or anaphylaxis)
Allergic infections such
   as aspergillosis or para-
   sites

▼ **Decreased IgE levels**
Agammaglobulinemia

notes

intravenous pyelography (IVP, Excretory urography [EUG], Intravenous urography [IUG, IVU])

Type of test X-ray with contrast dye

Normal findings

Normal size, shape, and position of the kidneys, renal pelvis, ureters, and bladder

Normal kidney excretory function as evidenced by the length of time for passage of contrast material through the kidneys

Test explanation

IVP is an x-ray study that uses radioopaque contrast material to visualize the kidneys, renal pelvis, ureters, and bladder. It is indicated on patients with:

1. Pain compatible with urinary stones
2. Blood in the urine
3. Proposed pelvic surgery to locate the ureters
4. Trauma to the urinary system
5. Urinary outlet obstruction
6. A suspected kidney tumor

If the artery leading to one of the kidneys is blocked, the dye cannot enter that kidney and the kidney will not be visualized. If the artery is partially blocked, the length of time required for the appearance of the contrast material will be prolonged.

With primary glomerular disease (e.g., glomerulonephritis), the glomerular filtrate is reduced, which causes a reduction in the quantity of dye filtered. As a result, kidney visualization is delayed. This indicates an estimate of renal function.

Defects in dye filling of the kidney can indicate renal tumors or cysts. Often intrinsic tumors, stones, extrinsic tumors, and scarring can partially or completely obstruct the flow of dye through the collecting system (pelvis, ureters, bladder). If the obstruction has been of sufficient duration, the collecting system proximal to the obstruction will be dilated (hydronephrosis). Retroperitoneal and pelvic tumors, aneurysms, and enlarged lymph nodes also can produce extrinsic compression and distortions of the opacified collecting system.

IVP is also used to assess the effect of trauma on the urinary system. Renal hematomas distort the renal contour. Renal artery laceration is suggested by nonopacification of one kidney. Laceration of the kidneys, pelvis, ureters, or bladder often causes

binding proteins. Therefore TIBC is an indirect yet accurate measurement of transferrin. *Ferritin* is not included in TIBC because it binds only stored iron. TIBC is increased in 70% of patients with iron deficiency.

Transferrin is a *negative* acute phase reactant protein. It is diminished in the face of acute inflammatory reactions, chronic illnesses such as malignancy, collagen vascular diseases, or liver diseases. Hypoproteinemia is also associated with reduced transferrin levels.

TIBC varies minimally according to iron intake. TIBC is more of a reflection of liver function (transferrin is produced by the liver) and nutrition than of iron metabolism. Transferrin values often are used to monitor the course of patients receiving hyperalimentation.

The percentage of transferrin and other mobile iron-binding proteins saturated with iron is calculated by dividing the serum iron level by the TIBC:

Transferrin saturation (TS) (%) = Serum iron level/TIBC × 100%

TS is decreased in patients with iron deficiency anemia. It is increased in patients with hemolytic, sideroblastic, or megaloblastic anemias. TS is also increased in patients with iron overload or poisoning. Increased intake or absorption of iron (as in hemochromatosis) leads to elevated iron levels. In such cases TIBC is unchanged; as a result, the percentage of transferrin saturation is very high.

Ferritin

The serum ferritin study is a good indicator of available iron stores in the body. Decreases in ferritin levels indicate a decrease in iron storage associated with iron deficiency anemia. The decrease in serum ferritin level often precedes other signs of iron deficiency such as decreased iron levels or changes in red blood cell size, chromasia, and number. Only when protein depletion is severe can ferritin be decreased by malnutrition. Increased levels are a sign of iron excess, as seen in hemochromatosis, hemosiderosis, iron poisoning, or recent blood transfusions. Increased ferritin is also noted in patients with megaloblastic anemia, hemolytic anemia, and chronic hepatitis. Ferritin is also used in patients with chronic renal failure to monitor iron stores.

A limitation of this study is that ferritin levels can also act as an "acute phase" reactant protein and may be elevated in conditions not reflecting iron stores (e.g., acute inflammatory diseases, infections, metastatic cancer, lymphomas).

Contraindication

- Patients with hemolytic diseases because they may have an artificially high iron content

Interfering factors

- Recent blood transfusions may affect test results.
- Recent ingestion of a meal containing high iron content may affect test results.
- Hemolytic diseases may be associated with an artificially high iron content.
- Recent administration of a radionuclide can cause abnormal levels if testing is performed by radioimmunoassay.

Procedure and patient care

Before

- Keep the patient fasting for 12 hours before the blood test. Water is permitted.

During

- Collect approximately 5 to 7 ml of venous blood in a red-top tube. The specimen should always be obtained using a 20-gauge or larger needle.
- Avoid hemolysis because the iron contained in the RBC will pour out into the serum and cause artificially high iron levels.

After

- Apply pressure to the venipuncture site.

Abnormal findings

▲ Increased serum iron levels	▼ Decreased serum iron levels
Hemosiderosis	Insufficient dietary iron
Hemochromatosis	Chronic blood loss
Hemolytic anemia	Inadequate absorption of iron
Hepatitis	Pregnancy (late)
Lead toxicity	Iron deficiency anemia
Iron poisoning	Neoplasia
Massive transfusion	Chronic bleeding

▲ **Increased TIBC levels**
Oral contraceptives
Pregnancy (late)
Polycythemia vera
Iron deficiency anemia

▼ **Decreased TIBC levels**
Hypoproteinemia
Inflammatory diseases
Cirrhosis
Hemolytic anemia
Pernicious anemia
Sickle cell anemia

▲ **Increased ferritin levels**
Hemochromatosis
Hemosiderosis
Megaloblastic anemia
Hemolytic anemia
Alcoholic/inflammatory
  hepatocellular disease
Inflammatory disease
Chronic illnesses (e.g.,
  leukemias, advanced
  cancers, cirrhosis,
  chronic hepatitis)
Collagen vascular dis-
  eases

▼ **Decreased ferritin levels**
Severe protein deficiency
Iron deficiency anemia
Hemodialysis

notes

lactate dehydrogenase (Lactic dehydrogenase [LDH])

Type of test Blood

Normal findings

Adult/elderly: 45-90 U/L (30° C), 115-225 IU/L, or 0.4-
   1.7 μmol/L (SI units)
Isoenzymes
   Adult/elderly:
      LDH-1: 17% to 27%
      LDH-2: 27% to 37%
      LDH-3: 18% to 25%
      LDH-4: 3% to 8%
      LDH-5: 0% to 5%
Child: 60-170 U/L (30° C)
Infant: 100-250 U/L
Newborn: 160-450 U/L

Test explanation

   LDH is found in the cells of many body tissues, especially the
heart, liver, red blood cells, kidneys, skeletal muscle, brain, and
lungs. The LDH is a measure of total LDH. There are actually five
separate fractions (isoenzymes) that make up the total LDH. Each
tissue contains a predominance of one or more LDH isoenzymes.

   In general, isoenzyme LDH-1 comes mainly from the heart;
LDH-2 comes primarily from the reticuloendothelial system;
LDH-3 comes from the lungs and other tissues; LDH-4 comes
from the kidney, placenta, and pancreas; and LDH-5 comes
mainly from the liver and striated muscle. In normal persons
LDH-2 makes up the greatest percentage of total LDH.

   With myocardial injury, the serum LDH level rises within 24
to 48 hours after a myocardial infarction (MI), peaks in 2 to 3
days, and returns to normal in approximately 5 to 10 days. This
makes the serum LDH level especially useful for a delayed diagnosis of patients with MI. In healthy individuals the LDH 2 fraction is greater than the LDH 1 fraction. Therefore the normal
LDH 1 to LDH 2 ratio is less than one. The reversal of the normal ratio (i.e., the ratio is greater than 1) is referred to as a
"flipped LDH." In an acute MI the flipped LDH ratio usually
appears in 12 to 24 hours.

   LDH is also measured in other body fluids. Elevated urine levels of total LDH indicate neoplasm or injury to the urologic sys-

tem. When the LDH in an effusion (pleural, cardiac or perito-neal) is >60% of the serum total LDH (i.e., effusion LDH/serum LDH ratio is greater than 0.6), the effusion is said to be an *exudate* and not a transudate.

Interfering factors

- Strenuous exercise may cause an elevation of total LDH and specifically LDH 1, 2, and 5
- Hemolysis of blood will cause false-positive LDH levels.
- ▼ Drugs that may cause *increased* LDH levels include alcohol, anesthetics, aspirin, and procainamide.

Procedure and patient care

Before

- Tell the patient that no fasting is required.
- Inform the patient if he or she will be receiving frequent venipuncture for the evaluation of an MI.

During

- Collect approximately 7 to 10 ml of venous blood in a red-top tube.
- Record the date and time when blood was drawn on the laboratory slip for an accurate evaluation of the temporal pattern of enzyme elevations.

After

- Apply pressure to the venipuncture site.

Abnormal findings

▲ **Increased values**
  Myocardial infarction
  Pulmonary disease (e.g., embolism, infarction, pneumonia, congestive heart failure)
  Hepatic disease (e.g., hepatitis, active cirrhosis, neoplasm)
  Red blood cell disease (e.g., hemolytic or megaloblastic anemia or red blood cell destruction from prosthetic heart valves)
  Skeletal muscle disease and injury (e.g., muscular dystro-phy, recent very strenuous exercises, or muscular trauma)
  Renal parenchymal disease (e.g., infarction, glomerulone-phritis, acute tubular necrosis, kidney transplantation rejection)
  Intestinal ischemia and infarction
  Testicular tumors (seminoma or dysgerminomas)

Lymphoma and other reticuloendothelial system tumors
Advanced solid tumor malignancies
Pancreatitis
Diffuse disease or injury (e.g., heat stroke, collagen
   disease, shock, hypotension)

notes

lipase

Type of test Blood

Normal findings 0-110 units/L or 0-417 U/L (SI units) (values are method dependent)

Test explanation

Because lipase was thought to be produced only in the pancreas, elevated serum levels were considered to be specific to pathologic pancreatic conditions (especially pancreatitis). It is now apparent that other conditions can be associated with elevated lipase levels. Lipase is excreted through the kidneys. Therefore elevated lipase levels are often found in patients with renal failure. Intestinal infarction or obstruction also can be associated with lipase elevation. However, the lipase elevations in nonpancreatic diseases are less than 3 times the upper limit of normal, as compared with pancreatitis, where they are often 5 to 10 times normal values. Still other conditions such as cholangitis, mumps, cholecystitis, or peptic ulcer are more rarely associated with elevated lipase levels.

In acute pancreatitis, elevated lipase levels usually parallel serum amylase levels. The lipase levels usually rise a little later than amylase (24 to 48 hours after the onset of pancreatitis) and remain elevated for 5 to 7 days.

Procedure and patient care

Before

- Instruct the patient to remain NPO, except for water, for 8 to 12 hours before the test.

During

- Collect 5 to 7 ml of venous blood in a red-top tube.
- Indicate on the laboratory slip drugs that may affect test results.

After

- Apply pressure to the venipuncture site.

Abnormal findings

Acute pancreatitis
Chronic relapsing pancreatitis
Pancreatic cancer

Pancreatic pseudocyst
Acute cholecystitis
Cholangitis
Extrahepatic duct obstruction
Renal failure
Bowel obstruction or infarction
Salivary gland inflammation or tumor
Peptic ulcer disease

notes

L

lipoproteins (High-density lipoprotein [HDL], Low-density lipoprotein [LDL], Very low–density lipoprotein [VLDL])

Type of test Blood

Normal findings

HDL
    Male: >45 mg/dl or >0.75 mmol/L (SI units)
    Female: >55 mg/dl or >0.91 mmol/L (SI units)
LDL: 60-180 mg/dl or <3.37 mmol/L (SI units)
VLDL: 25% to 50%

Test explanation

Lipoproteins are considered to be an accurate predictor of coronary heart disease (CHD). As part of the "lipid profile," these tests are performed to indicate persons at risk for developing heart disease and to monitor therapy if abnormalities are found. The "lipid profile" usually includes total cholesterol, triglycerides, HDL, LDL, and VLDL.

HDLs are carriers of cholesterol. It is suspected that the purpose of HDLs is to remove the cholesterol from the peripheral tissues and to transport this to the liver for excretion. Also, HDLs may have a protective effect by preventing cellular uptake of cholesterol and lipids. These potential actions may be the source of the protective cardiovascular characteristics associated with HDLs ("good cholesterol") within the blood. Both HDL and total cholesterol are independent variables of risk of CHD. When combined in a ratio fashion, the accuracy of prediction is increased. The total cholesterol/HDL ratio should be at least 5:1, with 3:1 being ideal.

LDLs are cholesterol rich. Cholesterol carried by LDLs can be deposited into the peripheral tissues and is associated with an increased risk of arteriosclerotic heart and vascular disease. Therefore high levels of LDL ("bad cholesterol") are atherogenic. LDL is most usually derived by subtracting the HDL plus one fifth of the triglycerides from the total cholesterol:

$$LDL = Total\ cholesterol - (HDL + Triglycerides/5)$$

There are other formulas for deriving LDL, which may account for different sets of normal values.

VLDLs, although carrying a small amount of cholesterol, are the predominant carriers of blood triglycerides. To a lesser degree, VLDLs are also associated with an increased risk of arteriosclerotic occlusive disease. The VLDL value is usually expressed as a percentage of total cholesterol. Levels in excess of 25% to 50% are associated with increased risk of coronary disease.

Interfering factors

- Smoking and alcohol ingestion decrease HDL levels.
- HDL values, like cholesterol, tend to significantly decrease for as long as 3 months following myocardial infarction.
- HDL is elevated in hypothyroid patients and diminished in hyperthyroid patients.

Procedure and patient care

Before

- Instruct the patient to fast for 12 to 14 hours before testing. Only water is permitted.
- Inform the patient that dietary indiscretion within the previous few weeks may influence lipoprotein levels.

During

- Collect 5 to 10 ml of venous blood in a red-top tube.

After

- Apply pressure to the venipuncture site.
- Instruct patients with high lipoprotein levels regarding diet, exercise, and appropriate body weight.

Abnormal findings

▲ **Increased HDL levels**
Familial HDL lipoproteinemia
Excessive exercise
Hypothyroidism

▼ **Decreased HDL levels**
Familial low HDL
Hepatocellular disease (e.g., hepatitis or cirrhosis)
Hypoproteinemia (e.g., nephrotic syndrome or malnutrition)

▲ **Increased LDL and VLDL**

Familiar LDL lipoproteinemia

Nephrotic syndrome

Glycogen storage diseases (e.g., von Gierke's disease)

Alcohol consumption

Chronic liver disease (e.g., hepatitis or cirrhosis)

Hepatoma

Gammopathies (e.g., multiple myeloma)

Familial hypercholestrolemia type IIa

Cushing's syndrome

Apoprotein CII deficiency

▼ **Decreased LDL and VLDL**

Familial hypolipoproteinemia

Hypoproteinemia (e.g., malabsorption, severe burns, or malnutrition)

Hyperthyroidism

notes

liver/spleen scanning (Liver scanning)

Type of test Nuclear scan

Normal findings Normal size, shape, and position of the liver and spleen

Test explanation

This radionuclide procedure is used to outline and detect structural changes of the liver and spleen. Because the scan can only demonstrate filling defects greater than 2 cm in diameter, false-negative results may occur in patients with space-occupying lesions (e.g., tumors, cysts, granulomas, abscesses) smaller than 2 cm. The liver scan can detect tumors, cysts, granulomas, abscesses, and diffuse infiltrative processes affecting the liver (e.g., amyloidosis, sarcoidosis).

Single Photon Emitting Computed Tomography (SPECT) has significantly improved the quality and accuracy of liver scanning. With SPECT scanning, the radionuclide is injected, and the scintillator is placed to receive images from multiple angles (around the circumference of the patient). This greatly increases the accuracy of nuclear liver scanning.

This scan can also identify portal hypertension. Normally most of the radionuclide administered during a liver scan is taken up by the liver. If the liver-to-spleen ratio is reversed (i.e., the spleen takes up more of the radionuclide), reversal of hepatic blood flow exists as a result of portal hypertension.

Splenic hematoma, abscess, cyst, tumor, infarction, and infiltrate processes such as granulomas can also be detected.

Contraindications

- Patients who are pregnant or lactating because of risk of damage to the fetus or infant.

Interfering factor

- Barium in the GI tract overlying the liver or spleen will produce defects on the scan that may be mistaken for masses.

Procedure and patient care

Before

- Tell the patient that no fasting or premedication is required.
- Assure the patient that he or she will not be exposed to large amounts of radiation because only tracer doses of isotopes are used.

During

- Note the following procedural steps:
  1. The patient is taken to the nuclear medicine department, where the radionuclide is administered intravenously.
  2. Thirty minutes after injection, a gamma ray detector is placed over the right upper quadrant of the patient's abdomen.
  3. The patient is placed in supine, lateral, and prone positions so that all surfaces of the liver can be visualized.
- Tell the patient that the only discomfort associated with this procedure is the IV injection of the radionuclide.

After

- Because only tracer doses of radioisotopes are used, inform the patient that no precautions need to be taken by others against radiation exposure.

Abnormal findings

Primary or metastatic tumor of the liver or spleen
Abscess of the liver or spleen
Hematoma of the liver or spleen
Hepatic or splenic cyst
Hemangioma
Lacerations of the liver or spleen
Infiltrative processes (e.g., sarcoidosis, amyloidosis, tuberculosis, or granuloma of the liver or spleen)
Cirrhosis
Portal hypertension
Accessory spleen
Splenic infarction

notes

lumbar puncture and cerebrospinal fluid examination (LP and CSF examination, Spinal tap, Spinal puncture, Cerebrospinal fluid analysis)

Type of test Fluid analysis

Normal findings

Pressure: less than 200 cm H_2O
Color: clear and colorless
Blood: none
Cells:
  RBC: 0
  WBC:
  Total
    Neonate: 0-30 cells/μl
    1-5 years: 0-20 cells/μl
    6-18 years: 0-10 cells/μl
    Adult: 0-5 cells/μl
  Differential
    Neutrophils: 0%-6%
    Lymphocytes: 40%-80%
    Monocytes: 15%-45%
Culture and sensitivity: no organisms present
Protein: 15-45 mg/dl CSF (up to 70 mg/dl in elderly adults
  and children)
Protein electrophoresis
  Prealbumin: 2%-7%
  Albumin: 56%-76%
  Alpha$_1$ globulin: 2%-7%
  Alpha$_2$ globulin: 4%-12%
  Beta globulin: 8% to 18%
  Gamma globulin: 3% to 12%
  Oligoclonal bands: none
  IgG: 0-4.5 mg/dl
Glucose: 50-75 mg/dl CSF or 60% to 70% of blood glucose
  level
Chloride: 700-750 mg/dl
Lactate dehydrogenase (LDH): <2-7.2 U/ml
Lactic acid: 10-25 mg/dl
Cytology: no malignant cells
Serology for syphilis: negative
Glutamine: 6-15 mg/dl

L

Test explanation

By placing a needle in the subarachnoid space of the spinal column, one can measure the pressure of that space and obtain CSF for examination and diagnosis. Lumbar puncture may also be used therapeutically to inject therapeutic or diagnostic agents and to administer spinal anesthetics.

Examination of the CSF includes evaluation for the presence of blood, bacteria, and malignant cells, along with quantification of the amount of glucose and protein present. Color is noted, and various other tests such as a serologic test for syphilis are performed.

Pressure

By attaching a sterile manometer to the needle used for LP, the pressure within the subarachnoid space can be measured. A pressure above 200 cm H_2O is considered abnormal and indicative of increased spinal pressure. Tumors, infection, hydrocephalus, and intracranial bleeding can cause increased intracranial and spinal pressure. Because the cranial venous sinuses are connected to the jugular veins, obstruction of those veins or the superior vena cava increases intracranial pressure.

Color

Normal CSF is clear and colorless. Color differences can occur with hyperbilirubinemia, hypercarotenemia, melanoma, or elevated proteins. A cloudy appearance may indicate an increase in the white blood cell (WBC) count or protein. A red tinge to the CSF indicates the presence of blood.

Blood

Normally, CSF contains no blood. Blood may be present because of bleeding into the subarachnoid space or because the needle used in the LP has inadvertently penetrated a blood vessel on the way into the subarachnoid space.

Cells

The number of red blood cells is merely an indication of the amount of blood present within the CSF. Except for a few lymphocytes, the presence of WBCs in the CSF is abnormal. The presence of polymorphonuclear leukocytes (neutrophils) is indicative of bacterial meningitis or cerebral abscess. When mononuclear leukocytes are present, viral or tubercular meningitis or encephalitis is suspected. Leukemia or other primary or metastatic malignant tumors may cause elevated WBCs.

Culture and sensitivity

The organisms that cause meningitis or brain abscess can be cultured from the CSF. A Gram stain of the CSF may give the clinician preliminary information about the causative infectious agent.

Protein

Normally, very little protein is found in CSF because protein is a large molecule that does not cross the blood-brain barrier. Diseases such as meningitis, encephalitis, or myelitis can alter the permeability of the blood-brain barrier, allowing protein to leak into the CSF. Furthermore, CNS tumors may produce and secrete protein into the CSF.

Glucose

The glucose level is decreased when the bacteria or cells within the CSF increase in number and catabolize the glucose. The cells may be inflammatory cells in response to infection or inflammation or cells that are shed by tumors.

Lactate dehydrogenase

Quantification of LDH (specifically fractions 4 and 5; see p. 173) is helpful in diagnosing bacterial meningitis. The source of LDH is the neutrophils that fight the invading bacteria. When the LDH level is elevated, infection or inflammation is suspected.

Lactic acid

Elevated levels indicate anaerobic metabolism associated with decreased oxygenation of the brain. CSF lactic acid is increased in both bacterial and fungal meningitis but not in viral meningitis.

Cytology

Examination of cells found in the CSF can determine if they are malignant.

Tumor markers

Increased levels of tumor markers such as carcinoembryonic antigen, alpha-fetoprotein, or human chorionic gonadotropin may indicate metastatic tumor.

Serology for syphilis

Latent syphilis is diagnosed by performing one of many presently available serologic tests on CSF. These include the Wasserman test, the Venereal Disease Research Laboratory (VDRL) test, and the fluorescent treponemal antibody (FTA) test.

Contraindications

- Patients with increased intracranial pressure
- Patients who have severe degenerative vertebral joint disease
- Patients with infection near the LP site

Potential complications

- Persistent CSF leak, causing severe headache
- Introduction of bacteria into CSF, causing suppurative meningitis
- Herniation of the brain through the tentorium cerebelli or herniation of the cerebellum through the foramen magnum
- Inadvertent puncture of the spinal cord caused by inappropriately high spinal puncture.
- Puncture of the aorta or vena cava, causing serious retroperitoneal hemorrhage

Procedure and patient care

Before

- Obtain informed consent if required by the institution.
- Perform a baseline neurologic assessment of the legs by assessing the patient's strengths, sensation, and movement.
- Tell the patient that no fasting or sedation is required.
- Instruct the patient to empty the bladder and bowels before the procedure.
- Explain to the patient that he or she must lie very still throughout this procedure.

During

- Note the following procedural steps:
    1. The patient is usually placed in the lateral decubitus (fetal) position.
    2. A local anesthetic is injected into the skin and subcutaneous tissues after the site has been aseptically cleaned.
    3. A spinal needle is placed through the skin and into the spinal canal. The subarachnoid space is entered.
    4. The needle is attached to a sterile manometer, and the pressure (opening pressure) is recorded.
    5. Three sterile test tubes are filled with 5 to 10 ml of CSF.
- Note that this procedure is performed by a physician in approximately 20 minutes.

After

- Apply digital pressure and an adhesive dressing to the puncture site.

- Place the patient in the prone position with a pillow under the abdomen to increase the intraabdominal pressure, which will indirectly increase the pressure in the tissues surrounding the spinal cord.
- Encourage the patient to drink increased amounts of fluid to replace the CSF removed during the lumbar puncture.
- Usually keep the patient in a reclining position for up to 12 hours to avoid the discomfort of potential postpuncture spinal headache.
- Assess the patient for numbness, tingling, and movement of the extremities; pain at the injection site; drainage of blood or CSF at the injection site; and the ability to void. Notify the physician of any unusual findings.

Abnormal findings

Brain neoplasm
Spinal cord neoplasm
Cerebral hemorrhage
Encephalitis
Myelitis
Tumor
Neurosyphilis
Degenerative brain disease
Autoimmune disorder
Hepatic encephalopathy
Coma
Meningitis
Viral or tubercular meningitis
Cerebral abscess
Degenerative cord or brain disease
Multiple sclerosis
Acute demyelinating polyneuropathy
Subarachnoid bleeding
Reye syndrome
Metastatic tumor

notes

lung scan (Pulmonary scintiphotography)

Type of test Nuclear scan

Normal findings Diffuse and homogeneous uptake of nuclear material by the lungs

Test explanation

This nuclear medicine procedure is used to identify defects in blood *perfusion* of the lung in patients with suspected pulmonary embolism. Blood flow to the lungs is evaluated using a macroaggregated albumin (MAA) tagged with technetium (Tc).

A homogeneous uptake of particles that fills the entire pulmonary vasculature conclusively rules out pulmonary embolism. If a defect in an otherwise smooth and diffusely homogeneous pattern is seen, a perfusion abnormality exists. This can indicate pulmonary embolism. Unfortunately, many other serious pulmonary parenchymal lesions (e.g., pneumonia, pleural fluid, emphysematous bullae) also cause a defect in pulmonary blood perfusion.

Contraindications

- Patients who are pregnant

Interfering factors

- Patients with known pulmonary parenchymal problems (e.g., pneumonia, emphysema, pleural effusion, tumors); these problems will give the picture of a perfusion defect and simulate pulmonary embolism.

Procedure and patient care

Before

- Tell the patient that no fasting is required.
- Note that a recent chest x-ray film should be available.

During

- Note the following procedural steps:
  1. The patient is given a peripheral IV injection of radionuclide-tagged MAA.
  2. While the patient lies in the appropriate position, a gamma ray detector is passed over the patient and records radionuclide uptake on Polaroid or x-ray film.

3. The patient is placed in the supine, prone, and various lateral positions, which allows for anterior, posterior, lateral, and oblique views, respectively.
- Tell the patient that no discomfort is associated with this test other than the peripheral venipuncture.

After
- Inform the patient that no radiation precautions are necessary.

Abnormal findings

Pulmonary embolism
Pneumonia
Tuberculosis
Emphysema
Tumor
Asthma
Atelectasis
Bronchitis
Chronic obstructive pulmonary disease

notes

Lyme disease test

Type of test Blood

Normal findings Negative (low titers of IgM and IgG antibodies)

Test explanation

Lyme disease is caused by a spirochete called *Borrelia burgdorferi*. The disease usually begins in the summer with a skin lesion called erythema chronicum migrans (ECM), which occurs at the site of a bite by a deer tick. Cultures of ECM can isolate the spirochete in half of the cases. However, it is hard to culture and takes a long time to grow. Currently, serologic studies are the most sensitive and specific tests for the detection of Lyme disease. These tests determine titers of specific immunoglobulin M (IgM) and specific IgG antibodies to the *B. burgdorferi* spirochete. Levels of specific IgM antibody peak during the third to sixth week after disease onset and then gradually decline.

Titers of specific IgG antibodies are generally low during the first several weeks of illness, reach maximal levels 4 to 6 months later, usually after the patient has developed arthritis, and often remain elevated for years. A single titer of specific IgM antibody may suggest the diagnosis. Acute and convalescent sera can be tested to verify the diagnosis.

Interfering factors

- Previous infection with *B. burgdorferi* can cause positive serologic testing.
- Other spirochete diseases (syphilis or leptospirosis) can cause false-positive results.

Procedure and patient care

Before
- Tell the patient that no fasting or special preparation is required.

During
- Collect approximately 7 to 10 ml of venous blood in a red-top tube.

After
- Apply pressure to the venipuncture site.

Abnormal finding

Lyme disease

notes

lymphangiography (Lymphangiogram, Lymphography)

Type of test X-ray with contrast dye

Normal findings Normal-sized lymph nodes containing no filling defects

Test explanation

Lymphangiography is especially useful in patients suspected of having lymphatic pathology (lymphoma or metastatic tumor). The test allows one to demonstrate the extent and level of lymphatic metastasis. The lymphangiogram is also useful in staging lymphoma patients and in evaluating the results of chemotherapy or radiation therapy. Because the contrast medium remains in the lymph nodes for 6 months to 1 year, repeat plain x-ray films may be done for continued follow-up of disease progression or response to treatment.

This test is also useful in the evaluation of patient with chronic leg swelling. Lack of flow of the dye into the pelvic lymphatic vessels indicates lymphatic vessel obstruction as the cause of the leg edema.

Contraindications

- Patients with an allergy to iodine dye or shellfish
- Patients with severe chronic lung diseases, cardiac disease, or advanced kidney or liver disease

Potential complications

- Lipoid (lipid) pneumonia
- Allergic reaction or allergy to iodine dye

Procedure and patient care

Before

- Obtain informed consent if required by the institution.
- Tell the patient that no fasting or sedation is required.
- Inform the patient that, if a blue-colored dye is used, he or she may note a bluish tinge in the urine. Excessive infiltration or IV administration of the lymphatic stain may create a transient bluish tint to a part of or the entire skin surface.

During

- Note the following procedural steps:
  1. A lymphatic stain is injected into the subcutaneous tissue between each of the first three toes in each foot to outline the lymphatic vessels.
  2. A small incision is made on the top of the foot (or hand).
  3. The lymphatic vessel is identified and cannulated.
  4. The dye is slowly infused into the vessel. Usually a low-rate infusion pump is used.
  5. The flow of iodine dye is followed by fluoroscopy.
  6. When the dye reaches the upper lumbar level, the flow of dye is discontinued.
  7. X-ray films are taken of the chest, abdomen, and pelvis to demonstrate the filling of the lymph nodes. Often the patient is asked to return in 24 hours to have additional x-ray studies done.
  8. On completion of the injection, the cannula is removed and the incision is sutured closed.
- Inform the patient that discomfort may be felt when the blue stain is injected subcutaneously and the feet are locally anesthetized.

After

- Observe the injection and incision sites for evidence of cellulitis. If the patient will be returning home, instruct him or her to evaluate the site for redness, pain, and swelling.
- Inform the patient that the sutures should be removed 7 to 10 days after the test.

Abnormal findings

Hodgkin's disease
Metastatic tumor involving the lymph glands
Lymphoma

notes

magnesium (Mg)

Type of test Blood

Normal findings
Adults: 1.2-2 mEq/L
Child: 1.4-1.7 mEq/L
Newborn: 1.4-2 mEq/L

Possible critical values <0.5 mEq/L or >3 mEq/L

Test explanation
Most of the magnesium is bound to an adenosine triphosphate (ATP) molecule, the main source of energy for the body. Therefore this electrolyte is critical in nearly all metabolic processes.

Low magnesium may increase cardiac irritability and aggravate cardiac arrhythmias. Hypermagnesemia retards neuromuscular conduction and is demonstrated as cardiac conduction slowing (widened PR and Q-T intervals with wide QRS).

Magnesium deficiency occurs in patients who are malnourished. Toxemia of pregnancy is also believed to be associated with reduced magnesium levels. Symptoms of magnesium depletion are mostly neuromuscular (i.e., weakness, irritability, tetany, electrocardiographic changes, delirium, and convulsions).

Increased magnesium levels most commonly are associated with ingestion of magnesium-containing antacids. Because most of the serum magnesium is excreted by the kidney, chronic renal diseases cause elevated magnesium levels. Symptoms of increased Mg include lethargy, nausea and vomiting, and slurred speech.

Interfering factors
- Hemolysis should be avoided when collecting this specimen.
- Drugs that *increase* magnesium levels include antacids, laxatives, calcium-containing medication, lithium, loop diuretics, and aminoglycosides antibiotics.

Procedure and patient care

Before
- Tell the patient that no special diet or fasting is required.

During
- Collect approximately 5 to 7 ml of venous blood in a red- or green-top tube.

- Avoid hemolysis.
- Indicate on the laboratory slip any drugs that may affect test results.

After
- Apply pressure to the venipuncture site.

Abnormal findings

▲ **Increased levels**
Renal insufficiency
Uncontrolled diabetes
Addison's disease
Hypothyroidism
Ingestion of magnesium-
    containing antacids or
    salts

▼ **Decreased levels**
Malnutrition
Malabsorption
Hypoparathyroidism
Alcoholism
Chronic renal disease
Diabetic acidosis

notes

magnetic resonance imaging (MRI, Nuclear magnetic resonance imaging [NMRI])

Type of test Magnetic field study

Normal findings No evidence of pathology

Test explanation

MRI has several advantages over computed tomography (CT) scanning, including the following:

1. MRI provides better contrast between normal tissue and pathologic tissue.
2. Obscuring bone artifacts that occur in CT scanning do not occur in MRI scanning.
3. Because rapidly flowing blood appears dark, which results from its quick motion, many blood vessels appear as dark lumens. This provides a natural contrast to the blood vessels when using MRI.
4. Because spatial information depends only on how the magnetic fields are varied in space, it is possible to image the transverse, sagittal, and coronal planes directly with MRI.

Although the full usefulness of MRI is yet to be determined, it shows promise in the evaluation of the following areas:

1. Head and surrounding structures
2. Spinal cord and surrounding structures
3. Face and surrounding structures
4. Neck
5. Mediastinum
6. Heart and great vessels
7. Liver
8. Kidney
9. Prostate
10. Bone and joints
11. Breast
12. Extremities and soft tissues

An important advantage of MRI imaging is that serial studies can be performed on the patient without any risk. This is useful in assessing the response of cancer to radiotherapy and chemotherapy. A major disadvantage of MRI is that patient eligibility is reduced as compared with CT scanning. For example, examination of patients requiring cardiac monitoring or having metal implants, metal joint replacements, pins for open reduction of fractures, pacemakers, or cerebral aneurysm clips will result in MRI image degradation and may endanger the patient.

Contraindications

- Patients who are extremely obese (over 300 pounds)
- Patients who are pregnant because the long-term effects of MRI are not known at this time
- Patients who are confused or agitated
- Patients who are unstable and require continuous life-support equipment because monitoring equipment cannot be used inside the scanner room
- Patients with implantable metal objects such as pacemakers, infusion pumps, aneurysm clips, inner ear implants, and metal fragments in one or both eyes because the magnet may move the object within the body and may injure the patient

Interfering factor

- Movement during the scan may cause artifacts on MRI.

Procedure and patient care

M

Before

- Obtain informed consent if required by the institution.
- Tell patients that they may read or talk to a child in the scanning room during the procedure because no risk of radiation from the procedure exists.
- Assess the patient for any contraindications for testing (e.g., aneurysm clips).
- If possible, show the patient a picture of the scanning machine and encourage verbalization of anxieties. Some patients may experience claustrophobia. Antianxiety medications may be helpful for those with mild claustrophobia.
- Instruct the patient to remove all metal objects (e.g., dental bridges, jewelry, hair clips, belts, credit cards) because they will create artifacts on the scan. The magnetic field can damage watches and credit cards. Also, movement of metal objects within the magnetic field can be detrimental to anyone within the field.
- Tell the patient that during the procedure he or she may hear a thumping sound. Earplugs are available if the patient wishes to use them.
- Inform the patient that no fluid or food restrictions are necessary before MRI.

- For comfort, instruct the patient to empty his or her bladder before the test.

During
- Note the following:
  1. The patient lies on a platform that slides into a tube containing the doughnut-shaped magnet. More recently, open magnets are available.
  2. The patient is instructed to lie very still during the procedure.
  3. During the scan, the patient can talk to and hear the staff via microphone or earphones placed in the scanner.
  4. A contrast medium may be injected intravenously.
- Note that this procedure is performed by a qualified radiologic technologist in approximately 30 to 90 minutes.

After
- Inform the patient that no special postprocedural care is needed.

Abnormal findings

Brain

Cerebral tumor
Cerebral infarction
Aneurysm
Arteriovenous malformation
Hemorrhage
Subdural hematoma
Multiple sclerosis

Other

Tumor (primary or metastatic)
Myocardial infarction
Atherosclerotic plaques
Aortic dissection
Aortic occlusion and stenosis
Abscess
Edema
Congenital heart disease
Dementia
Bone destructive lesion
Joint disorder
Degenerative vertebral disks

mammography (Mammogram)

Type of test X-ray

Normal findings

Class I: Negative
Class II: Benign
Class III: Benign—short-term follow-up suggested
Class IV: Suspicious—further evaluation suggested
Class V: Cancer highly suspected

Test explanation

Mammography is an x-ray examination of the breast used to identify cancers. In many cases, these cancers can be detected before they become palpable lesions.

Although mammography is not a substitute for breast biopsy, it is reliable and accurate when interpreted by a skilled radiologist. The accuracy of detection of breast cancer with mammography has been approximately 85%.

The American Cancer Society suggests that every woman over the age of 40 years should have a mammogram yearly.

Mammography can also detect other diseases of the breast. These include acute suppurative mastitis, abscess, fibrocystic changes, gross cysts, benign tumors (e.g., fibroadenoma), and intraglandular lymph nodes.

A women receives minimal radiation exposure during mammography (about 0.5 rads per view). Most mammograms include two views of each breast.

Contraindications

- Patients who are pregnant because of the risk of fetal damage
- Women under the age of 25 years

Interfering factors

- Talc powder can give the impression of calcification within the breast.
- Jewelry worn around the neck can preclude total visualization of the breast.
- Breast augmentation implants prevent total visualization of the breast.
- Previous breast surgery can alter or distort the mammogram findings.

M

Procedure and patient care

Before

- Inform the patient that some discomfort may be experienced during breast compression. This compression allows better visualization of the breast tissue. Assure the patient that the breast will not be harmed by the compression.
- Tell the patient that no fasting is required.
- Explain to the patient that a minimal radiation dose will be used during the test.

During

- Note the following procedural steps:
  1. The patient is taken to the radiology department and seated in front of a mammogram machine.
  2. One breast is placed on the x-ray plate.
  3. The x-ray cone is brought down on the top of the breast to compress it gently between the broadened cone and the x-ray plate.
  4. The x-ray film is exposed. This is the craniocaudal view.
  5. The x-ray plate is turned about 45 degrees and placed on the inner aspect of the breast. This creates the mediolateral view.

After

- Take this opportunity to instruct the patient in breast self-examination.

Abnormal findings

Breast cancer
Benign tumor (e.g., fibroadenoma)
Breast cyst
Fibrocystic changes
Breast abscess
Suppurative mastitis

notes

obstruction series

Type of test X-ray

Normal findings
No evidence of bowel obstruction
No abnormal calcifications
No free air

Test explanation
The obstruction series is a group of x-ray films performed on the abdomen of patients with suspected bowel obstruction, paralytic ileus, perforated viscus, abdominal abscess, kidney stones, appendicitis, or foreign body ingestion. This series of films usually consists of at least two x-ray studies. The first is an *erect abdominal* film that should include visualization of both diaphragms. The film is examined for evidence of free air under either diaphragm, which is pathognomonic for a perforated viscus. This view is also used to detect air-fluid levels within the intestine; the presence of an air-fluid level is compatible with bowel obstruction or paralytic ileus. Occasionally patients are too ill to stand erect. In this case, an x-ray film can be taken with the patient in the left lateral decubitus position. If free air is present, it will be seen between the liver and the right side of the abdominal wall. As with the erect-position film, air-fluid levels also can be detected.

The second view in the obstruction series is usually a *supine abdominal* x-ray study. This is very similar to the kidney, ureter, and bladder (KUB) x-ray study. An abdominal abscess may be seen as a cluster of tiny bubbles within one localized area. A calcification within the course of the ureter could indicate a kidney ureteral stone. A small calcification in the right lower quadrant on the film of a patient complaining of pain in this quadrant may be an appendicolith. A gas-filled, distended bowel is compatible with bowel obstruction or paralytic ileus. The obstruction series can also be used to monitor the clinical course of patients with gastrointestinal (GI) disease.

Frequently a *cross-table lateral* view of the abdomen is included in an obstruction series to detect abdominal aorta calcification, which often occurs in older patients. The calcification represents the anterior wall of the aorta. If an aortic aneurysm exists, this calcification will be seen to protrude from the spine.

O

A *supine abdominal* x-ray study can be used as a "scout film" before performing GI or abdominal x-ray studies that use contrast, such as a barium enema or intravenous pyelogram.

Contraindications

- Patients who are pregnant

Interfering factor

- Previous GI barium contrast study

Procedure and patient care

Before
- Ensure that all radiopaque clothing has been removed.

During
- Although the procedure varies from facility to facility, note that usually a supine abdominal x-ray film, erect abdominal film, and perhaps a lower erect chest film are taken. Often a cross-table lateral x-ray film is also included.

After
- Note that no special aftercare is needed.

Abnormal findings

Kidney stone
Bowel obstruction
Organomegaly
Presence of a foreign body
Bladder distention
Abdominal abscess
Perforated viscus
Abdominal aortic calcification
Appendicolithiasis
Paralytic ileus
Abdominal aortic aneurysm
Peritoneal effusion/ascites
Abnormal position of the kidneys
Soft tissue masses

notes

OSMOLALITY

osmolality, serum
osmolality, urine

Type of test Blood, urine

Normal findings

Serum:
Adult/elderly: 285-295 mOsm/kg H_2O
Urine:
Random specimen: 50-1400 mOsm/kg H_2O, depending on
  fluid intake (SI units)

Possible critical values

Serum:
<265 mOsm/kg H_2O
>320 mOsm/kg H_2O
Urine:
<100 mOsm/kg H_2O in overhydration
>800 mOsm/kg H_2O in dehydration

Test explanation

O

  Osmolality measures the concentration of dissolved particles in
blood or urine. As the amount of free water increases or the
amount of particles decreases, osmolality decreases. As the
amount of water decreases or the amount of particles increases,
osmolality increases. Osmolality increases with dehydration and
decreases with overhydration.
  Urine osmolality is used in the precise evaluation of the concentrating ability of the kidney. Osmolality is also useful in evaluating fluid and electrolyte imbalance. The test is very helpful in
the evaluation of seizures, ascites, hydration status, acid-base balance, and suspected ADH abnormalities. Osmolality is also helpful in identifying the presence of organic acids, sugars, or ethanol.
In these cases there is an *osmolal gap*. This gap represents the difference between what the osmolality should be (based on calculations of serum sodium, glucose and BUN—the three most important solutes in the blood) and the osmolality as truly
measured. If the "gap" is large, the presence of solutes such as
organic acids (ketones), unusually high levels of glucose, or ethanol by-products is suspected.

Procedure and patient care

Before

- Inform the patient that preparation for a fasting urine specimen may require a high-protein diet for 3 days before the test. Instruct the patient to eat a dry supper the evening before the test and to drink no fluids until the test is completed the next morning. Normally, however, no fasting is required.

During

Serum

- Collect approximately 5 to 10 ml of venous blood in a red-top tube.
- For pediatric patients, draw blood from a heel stick.

Urine

- Collect a first-voided urine specimen for a random sample.
- For a fasting specimen, instruct the patient to empty the bladder at approximately 6 AM and to discard the urine. Collect the test urine at 8 AM.

After

- Apply pressure to the venipuncture site.

Abnormal findings

▲ **Increased serum osmolality**

Hypernatremia
Dehydration
Hyperglycemia
Azotemia/uremia
Hyperosmolar nonketotic hyperglycemia
Diabetes insipidus
Hypercalcemia
Renal tubular necrosis
Shock

▼ **Decreased serum osmolality**

Hyponatremia
Overhydration
Syndrome of inappropriate antidiuretic hormone secretion (SIADH)

▲ **Increased urine osmolality**
Syndrome of inappropriate antidiuretic hormone secretion (SIADH)
Acidosis
Shock
Hypernatremia
Hepatic cirrhosis
Congestive heart failure
Addison's disease

▼ **Decreased urine osmolality**
Diabetes insipidus
Hypercalcemia
Excess fluid intake
Renal tubular necrosis
Aldosteronism
Hypokalemia

notes

O

oximetry (Pulse oximetry, Ear oximetry, Oxygen saturation)

Type of test Photodiagnostic

Normal findings ≥95%

Possible critical values ≤75%

Test explanation

Oximetry is a noninvasive method of monitoring arterial blood oxygen saturation (SaO_2). The SaO_2 is the ratio of oxygenated hemoglobin to the total amount of hemoglobin. The SaO_2 is expressed as a percentage; for example, a saturation of 95% indicates that 95% of the total hemoglobin attachments for oxygen have oxygen attached to them.

Oximetry is typically used for monitoring the patient's oxygenation status during the perioperative period (or any time of heavy sedation) and for patients receiving mechanical ventilation. This test is also frequently used in many clinical situations, such as pulmonary rehabilitation programs, stress testing, and sleep laboratories. This test is commonly used to titrate levels of oxygen in hospitalized patients.

Procedure and patient care

Before
- Tell the patient that no fasting is required.

During
- Rub the patient's earlobe, pinna (upper part of the ear), or fingertip to increase blood flow.
- Clip the monitoring probe or sensor to the ear or finger.
- Note that this study is usually performed by a respiratory therapist or nurse at the patient's bedside in a few minutes.

After
- Note that no special aftercare is needed.

Abnormal findings

▲ **Increased levels**
Increased inspired O_2
Hyperventilation

▼ **Decreased levels**
Inadequate O_2 in inspired air
Hypoxic lung diseases
Hypoxic cardiac diseases
Severe hypoventilation states

Papanicolaou smear (Pap smear, Pap test, Cytologic test for cancer)

Type of test Microscopic examination

Normal findings No abnormal or atypical cells

Test explanation

A Pap smear is taken to detect neoplastic cells in cervical and vaginal secretions. This test is based on the fact that normal cells and abnormal cervical and endometrial neoplastic cells are shed into the cervical and vaginal secretions. By examining these secretions microscopically, one can detect early cellular changes compatible with premalignant conditions or an existing malignant condition. The Pap smear is 95% accurate in detecting cervical carcinoma; however, its accuracy in detection of endometrial carcinoma is only approximately 40%.

Reports are in terms of cervical intraepithelial neoplasia (CIN). This is a simple designation of the spectrum of intraepithelial dysplasia, which usually occurs before invasive cervical cancer. The subclasses of CIN are defined as follows:

CIN 1: mild and mild-to-moderate dysplasia
CIN 2: moderate and moderate-to-severe dysplasia
CIN 3: severe dysplasia and carcinoma in situ

Most recently, the Bethesda System for reporting cervical/vaginal cytologic diagnoses was developed and revised by the National Cancer Institute. This system includes evaluation of the following:

Adequacy of specimen
General categorization (optional)
Descriptive diagnosis
Epithelial cell abnormalities (squamous and glandular cells)

A Pap smear also may be performed to follow some abnormalities (e.g., infertility). An abnormal maturation index (MI) is characteristic of an estrogen-progesterone imbalance. The MI is calculated by determining the ratio of parabasal cervical cells to intermediate cells to superficial cells. The normal ovulating adult MI is 0/70/30. The MI is used more frequently for determination of menstrual status and ovarian function.

Pap smears should be part of the routine pelvic examination, which is usually performed once a year on women over 18 years of age (or even earlier when the patient is sexually active).

P

Contraindications

- Patients presently having routine normal menses because this can alter test interpretation.
- Patients with vaginal infections.

Interfering factors

- A delay in fixing a specimen allows the cells to dry, destroys effectiveness of the stain, and makes cytologic interpretation difficult.
- Using lubricating jelly on the speculum can alter the specimen.
- Douching and tub bathing may wash away cellular deposits and interfere with the test results.
- Menstrual flow may alter test results.
- Infections may interfere with hormonal cytology.

Procedure and patient care

Before

- Instruct the patient not to douche or tub bathe during the 24 hours before the Pap smear. (Some physicians prefer that patients refrain from sexual intercourse for 24 to 48 hours before the test.)
- Instruct the patient to empty her bladder before the examination.
- Tell the patient that no fasting or sedation is required.

During

- Note the following procedural steps:
  1. The patient is placed in the lithotomy position.
  2. A vaginal speculum is inserted to expose the cervix.
  3. Material is collected from the cervical canal by rotating a moist, saline cotton swab or spatula within the cervical canal and in the squamocolumnar junction.
  4. The cells are immediately wiped across a clean glass slide and fixed either by immersing the slide in equal parts of 95% alcohol and ether or by using a commercial spray (e.g., Aqua Net hair spray).
  5. The slide is labeled with the patient's name, age, and parity and with the date of her last menstrual period.

After

- Inform the patient that usually she will be notified of results.

Abnormal findings

Cancer
Infertility
Venereal disease
Reactive inflammatory changes
Fungal infection
Parasitic infection
Herpes infection

notes

paracentesis (Peritoneal fluid analysis, Abdominal paracentesis, Ascitic fluid cytology, Peritoneal tap)

Type of test Fluid analysis

Normal findings

Gross appearance: Clear, serous, light yellow, <50 ml
Red blood cells (RBCs): None
White blood cells (WBCs): <300/μl
Protein: <4.1 g/dl
Glucose: 70-100 mg/dl
Amylase: 138-404 U/L
Lactate dehydrogenase (LDH): Similar to serum lactate dehydrogenase
Cytology: No malignant cells
Bacteria: None
Fungi: None

Test explanation

Paracentesis is an invasive procedure entailing the insertion of a needle or catheter into the peritoneal cavity for removal of ascitic fluid for diagnostic and therapeutic purposes.

Diagnostically, paracentesis is performed to obtain and analyze fluid to determine the etiology of the peritoneal effusion. Peritoneal fluid is classified as to whether it is a transudate or exudate. This is an important differentiation and is very helpful in determining the etiology of the effusion. *Transudates* are most frequently caused by congestive heart failure, cirrhosis, nephrotic syndrome, myxedema, peritoneal dialysis, and hypoproteinemia. *Exudates* are most often found in infectious or neoplastic conditions. However, collagen vascular disease, gastrointestinal diseases, trauma, and drug hypersensitivity also may cause an exudative effusion.

Therapeutically this procedure is done to remove large amounts of fluid from the abdominal cavity. Usually these patients experience transient relief of symptoms (shortness of breath, distention, and early satiety) because of the fluid within the abdominal cavity.

The peritoneal fluid is usually evaluated for gross appearance, RBCs, WBCs, protein, glucose, amylase, ammonia, alkaline phosphatase, LDH, cytology, bacteria, fungi, and other tests such as CEA levels. Each is discussed separately. Urea and creatinine may be measured if there is a question whether the fluid may represent urine from a perforated bladder.

Gross appearance

Transudative peritoneal fluid may be clear, serous, and light yellow, especially in patients with hepatic cirrhosis. Milk-colored peritoneal fluid may result from the escape of chyle from blocked abdominal or thoracic lymphatic ducts. Conditions that may cause lymphatic blockage include lymphoma, carcinoma, and tuberculosis involving the abdominal or thoracic lymph nodes. The triglyceride value in a chylous effusion exceeds 110 mg/dl.

Exudative fluid is cloudy or turbid fluid. Bloody fluid may be the result of a traumatic tap (the aspirating needle penetrates a blood vessel), intraabdominal bleeding, tumor, or hemorrhagic pancreatitis. Bile-stained, green fluid may result from a ruptured gallbladder, acute pancreatitis, or perforated intestines.

Cell counts

Normally no RBCs should be present. The presence of RBCs may indicate neoplasms, tuberculosis, or intraabdominal bleeding. Increased WBC counts may be seen with peritonitis, cirrhosis, and tuberculosis.

Protein count

Total protein levels greater than 3 g/dl are characteristic of *exudates*, whereas *transudates* usually have a protein content of less than 3 g/dl. It is now thought that the *albumin gradient* between serum and ascitic fluid can differentiate better between the transudate and exudate nature of ascites than can the total protein content. This gradient is obtained by subtracting the ascitic albumin value from the serum albumin value. Values of 1.1 g/dl or more suggest a transudate, and values less than 1.1 g/dl suggest an exudate. The total protein ratio (fluid/serum) has been used to differentiate exudate from transudate. A total protein ratio of fluid to serum of greater than 0.5 is considered to be an exudate.

Glucose

Usually peritoneal glucose levels approximate serum glucose levels. Decreased levels may indicate tuberculous/bacterial peritonitis or peritoneal carcinomatosis.

Amylase

Increased amylase levels may be seen in patients with pancreatic trauma; pancreatic pseudocyst; acute pancreatitis; and intes-

P

tinal necrosis, perforation, or strangulation. In these diseases the amylase level is usually >1.5 times higher than serum levels.

Bacteria

Usually the fluid is cultured, and the antibiotic sensitivities are determined. Gram stains are often performed.

Gram stain and bacteriologic culture

The presence of bacteria may indicate intraabdominal infection. Culture and Gram stains identify the organisms involved in the infection.

Fungi

Fungi may indicate infections with histoplasmosis, candidiasis, or coccidioidomycosis.

Contraindications

- Patients with coagulation abnormalities or bleeding tendencies
- Patients with only a small amount of fluid or extensive previous abdominal surgery

Potential complications

- Hypovolemia if a large volume of peritoneal fluid is removed
- Peritonitis

Procedure and patient care

Before

- Obtain informed consent for this procedure.
- Tell the patient that no fasting or sedation is necessary.
- Have the patient urinate or empty the bladder before the test. This will help to prevent accidental bladder trauma.
- Measure abdominal girth.
- Obtain the patient's weight.
- Obtain baseline vital signs.

During

- Note the following procedural steps:
  1. Position the person in a high Fowler's position in bed.
  2. The needle insertion site is aseptically cleansed and anesthetized locally.
  3. A scalpel may be used to make a stab wound in the skin to allow the cannula or needle to enter.
  4. A trocar, cannula, or needle is threaded through the incision.

5. Tubing is attached to the cannula. The other end of the tubing is placed in the collection receptacle (usually a container with a pressurized vacuum).

After

- All tests performed on peritoneal fluid should be performed immediately to avoid false results due to chemical or cellular deterioration.
- Place a small bandage over the needle site.
- Label the specimen with the patient's name, date, source of fluid, and diagnosis.
- Observe the puncture site for bleeding, continued drainage, or signs of inflammation.
- Measure the abdominal girth and weight of the patient; compare with baseline values.
- Monitor vital signs for evidence of hemodynamic changes. Watch for signs of hypotension if a large volume of fluid is removed.

Abnormal findings

Exudate

Lymphoma
Carcinoma
Tuberculosis
Peritonitis
Pancreatitis
Ruptured viscus

Transudate

Hepatic cirrhosis
Portal hypertension
Nephrotic syndrome
Hypoproteinemia
Congestive heart failure
Abdominal trauma
Peritoneal bleeding

notes

partial thromboplastin time, activated (APTT, Partial thromboplastin time [PTT])

Type of test Blood

Normal findings

APTT: 30-40 seconds
PTT: 60-70 seconds
Patients receiving anticoagulant therapy: 1.5-2.5 times control value in seconds

Possible critical values

APTT: >70 seconds
PTT: >100 seconds

Test explanation

The PTT test is used to assess the intrinsic system and the common pathway of clot formation. PTT evaluates factors I (fibrinogen), II (prothrombin), V, VIII, IX, X, XI, and XII. When any of these factors exists in inadequate quantities, as in hemophilia A and B or consumptive coagulopathy, the PTT is prolonged. Because factors II, IX, and X are vitamin K–dependent factors, biliary obstruction, which precludes gastrointestinal absorption of fat and fat-soluble vitamins (e.g., vitamin K), can reduce their concentration and thus prolong the PTT. Because coagulation factors are made in the liver, hepatocellular diseases will also prolong the PTT. The appropriate dose of heparin can be monitored by the PTT.

Recently activators have been added to the PTT test reagents to shorten normal clotting time and provide a narrow normal range. This shortened time is called the *activated* PTT (APTT). The normal APTT is 30 to 40 seconds. Desired ranges for therapeutic anticoagulation are 1.5 to 2.5 times normal (e.g., 70 seconds). The APTT specimen should be drawn 30 to 60 minutes before the patient's next heparin dose is given.

Procedure and patient care

Before

- If the patient is receiving heparin by intermittent injection, plan to draw the blood specimen for the APTT 30 minutes to 1 hour before the next dose of heparin.

During

- Collect 5 to 14 ml of venous blood in one or two blue-top tubes.

After

- Apply pressure to the venipuncture site. Remember, if the patient is receiving anticoagulants or has coagulopathies, the bleeding time will be increased.

Abnormal findings

▲ **Increased levels**
Acquired or congenital clotting factor deficiencies
Cirrhosis of the liver
Vitamin K deficiency
Leukemia
Disseminated intravascular coagulation
Heparin administration
Hypofibrinogenemia
von Willebrand's disease
Hemophilia

▼ **Decreased levels**
Early stages of disseminated intravascular coagulation
Extensive cancer

P

notes

---

pelvic/rectal ultrasonography (Obstetric echography, Pregnant uterus ultrasonography, Pelvic ultrasonography in pregnancy, Obstetric ultrasonography, Vaginal ultrasound, Prostate ultrasound)

Type of test   Ultrasound

Normal findings

Normal fetal and placental size and position
Normal pelvic organs
Normal prostate

Test explanation

Pelvic ultrasonography may be useful in the *obstetric patient* to diagnose the following circumstances:

1. Making an early diagnosis of normal pregnancy or abnormal pregnancy (e.g., tubal pregnancy)
2. Identifying multiple pregnancies
3. Differentiating a tumor (e.g., hydatidiform mole) from a normal pregnancy
4. Determining the age of the fetus by the diameter of the head.
5. Measuring the rate of fetal growth
6. Identifying placental abnormalities such as placenta previa
7. Determining the position of the placenta for amniocentesis.
8. Determining fetal position
9. Identifying an ectopic pregnancy

Pelvic ultrasound is used in the *nonpregnant woman* to monitor the endometrium in patients who take tamoxifen and to aid in the diagnosis of:

1. Ovarian cyst
2. Ovarian tumor
3. Tubo-ovarian abscess
4. Uterine fibroids
5. Uterine cancer
6. Pelvic inflammatory disease (PID)
7. Thickened uterine endometrium (stripe) (caused by cancer, hyperplasia, etc.)

In men, rectal ultrasound of the prostate is a very valuable tool in the early diagnosis of prostate cancer. When combined with rectal digital examination and prostate-specific antigen (see p.

277), very small prostate cancers can be identified. Prostate/rectal sonography is also helpful in evaluating the seminal vesicles and other perirectal tissue. Ultrasound is used to guide the direction of a prostate biopsy and can be extremely helpful in quantitating the volume of prostate cancer. When radiation therapy implantation is required for treatment, ultrasound is used to map the exact location of the prostate cancer. Rectal ultrasound is very helpful in staging rectal cancers as well. The depth of transmural involvement and presence of extrarectal extension can be accurately assessed.

Pelvic/rectal ultrasonography can be performed with the transducer placed on the anterior abdomen or in the vagina or rectum with a specially designed vaginal probe.

Contraindications

- Patients with latex allergy (rectal/vaginal probes require the use of a latex condom-like sac)

Interfering factors

- Patients who have had recent gastrointestinal (GI) contrast studies because barium creates severe distortion of reflective sound waves
- Patients with air-filled bowels because gas does not transmit sound waves well
- Failure to fill the bladder which may make identification of pelvic organs difficult

Procedure and patient care

Before

- Explain the procedure to the patient.
- For pelvic ultrasound, give the patient three to four glasses (200 to 350 ml) of water or other liquid 1 hour before the examination and instruct the patient *not* to void until after the procedure is completed. This will permit visualization of the bladder, which is used as a reference point in pelvic anatomy. This is not required for vaginal/rectal ultrasound.
- If a transabdominal ultrasound is required urgently and there is no time to fill the bladder by ingestion or administration of fluids, a bladder catheter is inserted, and the bladder is filled with water.
- Tell the patient that no fasting or sedation is required.
- Instruct the patient that a small-volume rectal enema is required approximately 1 hour before a rectal ultrasound.

During

Note the following procedural steps:

- The ultrasonographer applies a greasy, conductive paste to the abdomen to enhance sound transmission and reception.
- A transducer is passed vertically and horizontally over the skin.
- If a vaginal probe is used, it is inserted via the vagina and angled to identify the various parts of the pelvis.
- A digital rectal examination may be performed before rectal ultrasound to ensure complete evacuation of stool.
- A draped and lubricated ultrasound probe is placed within the rectum.

After

- Remove the lubricant from the patient's skin.
- Provide an opportunity for the patient to void and cleanse the perineal area.

Abnormal findings

Tubal pregnancy
Abdominal pregnancy
Hydatidiform mole
Intrauterine growth retardation
Multiple fetuses
Fetal death
Abnormal fetal position (e.g., breech, transverse)
Placenta previa
Polyhydramnios
Neoplasm of the ovaries, uterus, or fallopian tubes
Cysts
Abscesses
Hydrocephalus of the fetus
Intrauterine device localization
Prostate cancer
Benign prostatic hypertrophy
Prostatitis
Seminal vesicle tumor
Prostate abscess
Perirectal abscess
Intrarectal or perirectal tumor

phosphate (P, PO₄, Inorganic phosphorus)

Type of test Blood

Normal findings

Adult: 3-4.5 mg/dl or 0.97-1.45 mmol/L (SI units)
Elderly: values slightly lower than adult
Child: 4.5-6.5 mg/dl or 1.45-2.1 mmol/L (SI units)
Newborn: 4.3-9.3 mg/dl or 1.4-3 mmol/L (SI units)

Possible critical values <1 mg/dl

Test explanation

Only a small part of total body phosphate is inorganic phosphate (i.e., not part of another organic compound). It is the *inorganic* phosphate that is measured when one requests a "phosphate," "phosphorus," "inorganic phosphorus," or "inorganic phosphate." Most of the body's inorganic phosphorus is combined with calcium within the skeleton; however, approximately 15% of the phosphorus exists in the blood as a phosphate salt.

Interfering factors

- Laxatives or enemas containing sodium phosphate can increase phosphorus levels.
- Recent carbohydrate ingestion, including IV glucose administration, causes decreased phosphorus levels because phosphorus enters the cell with glucose.

Procedure and patient care

Before

- Keep the patient NPO after midnight on the day of the test.
- If indicated, discontinue IV fluids with glucose for several hours before the test.

During

- Collect approximately 5 to 10 ml of venous blood in a red-top tube.
- Avoid hemolysis. Handle the tube carefully.
- Use a heel stick to draw blood from infants.

After

- Apply pressure to the venipuncture site.

P

Abnormal findings

▲ **Increased levels (hyperphosphatemia)**
Renal failure
Increased dietary or IV intake of phosphorus
Acromegaly
Hypoparathyroidism
Bone metastasis
Sarcoidosis
Hypocalcemia
Liver disease
Renal failure
Acidosis
Rhabdomyolysis
Advanced lymphoma or myeloma
Hemolytic anemia

▼ **Decreased levels (hypophosphatemia)**
Inadequate dietary ingestion of phosphorus
Chronic antacid ingestion
Hyperparathyroidism
Hypercalcemia
Chronic alcoholism
Vitamin D deficiency
Diabetic acidosis
Hyperinsulinism
Rickets (childhood)
Osteomalacia (adult)
Malnutrition
Alkalosis
Sepsis

notes

platelet count (Thrombocyte count)

Type of test Blood

Normal findings

Adult/elderly: 150,000-400,000/mm^3 or 150 to 400 × 10^9/L (SI units)
Premature infant: 100,000-300,000/mm^3
Newborn: 150,000-300,000/mm^3
Infant: 200,000-475,000 mm^3
Child: 150,000-400,000/mm^3

Possible critical values <50,000 or >1 million/mm^3

Test explanation

The platelet count is an actual count of the number of platelets (thrombocytes) per cubic milliliter of blood. It is performed on all patients who develop petechiae (small hemorrhages in the skin), spontaneous bleeding, or increasingly heavy menses, or it is used to monitor the course of the disease or therapy for thrombocytopenia or bone marrow failure.

Platelet activity is essential to blood clotting. Counts of 150,000 to 400,000/mm^3 are considered normal. Counts less than 100,000/mm^3 are considered to indicate *thrombocytopenia;* *thrombocytosis* is said to exist when counts are greater than 400,000/mm^3. *Thrombocythemia* is a term used to indicate a platelet count in excess of 1 million/mm^3. The most common associative disease with spontaneous thrombocytosis is malignancy (leukemia, lymphoma, or solid tumors, such as colon). Thrombocytosis may also occur with polycythemia vera and postsplenectomy syndromes.

Causes of thrombocytopenia (decreased number of platelets) include the following:

1. Reduced production of platelets (secondary to bone marrow failure or infiltration of fibrosis, tumor, etc.)
2. Sequestration of platelets (secondary to hypersplenism)
3. Accelerated destruction of platelets (secondary to antibodies, infections, drugs, prosthetic heart valves)
4. Consumption of platelets (secondary to disseminated intravascular coagulation)
5. Platelet loss from hemorrhage

P

6. Dilution, with large volume, of blood transfusions that contain very few, if any, platelets

Interfering factors

- Living in high altitudes may cause increased platelet levels.
- Because platelets can clump together, automated counting is subject to at least a 10% to 15% error.
- Strenuous exercise may cause increased levels.
- Drugs that may cause *increased* levels include oral contraceptives.
- Drugs that may cause *decreased* levels include chemotherapeutic agents, colchicine, hydralazine, indomethacin, isoniazid (INH), quinidine, thiazide diuretics, and tolbutamide (Orinase).

Procedure and patient care

Before
- Tell the patient that no fasting is required.

During
- Collect approximately 5 to 7 ml of peripheral venous blood in a lavender-top tube.
- List on the laboratory slip any drugs or other factors that may affect test results.

After
- Apply pressure to the venipuncture site.

Abnormal findings

▲ **Increased levels (thrombocytosis)**
Malignant disorder
Polycythemia vera
Postsplenectomy syndrome
Rheumatoid arthritis
Iron deficiency anemia

▼ **Decreased levels (thrombocytopenia)**
Hypersplenism
Hemorrhage
Immune thrombocytopenia
Leukemia and other myelofibrosis disorders
Thrombotic thrombocytopenia
Inherited thrombocytopenia disorders (e.g., Wiskott-Aldrich, Bernard Soulier, or Zieve syndromes)
Disseminated intravascular coagulation

Systemic lupus erythemato-
sus
Pernicious anemia
Hemolytic anemia
Cancer chemotherapy
Infection

notes

P

potassium, blood (K⁺)

Type of test Blood

Normal findings

Adults/elderly: 3.5-5 mEq/L or 3.5-5 mmol/L (SI units)
Child: 3.4-4.7 mEq/L
Infant: 4.1-5.3 mEq/L
Newborn: 3.9-5.9 mEq/L

Possible critical values

Adult: <2.5 or >6.5 mEq/L
Newborn: <2.5 or >8 mEq/L

Test explanation

Potassium is the major cation within the cell. Symptoms of *hyperkalemia* include irritability, nausea, vomiting, intestinal colic, and diarrhea. The electrocardiogram may demonstrate peaked T waves, a widened QRS complex, and depressed ST segment. Signs of *hypokalemia* are related to a decrease in contractility of smooth, skeletal, and cardiac muscles, which results in weakness, paralysis, hyporeflexia, ileus, increased cardiac sensitivity to digoxin, cardiac arrhythmias, flattened T waves, and prominent U waves. This electrolyte has profound effects on the heart rate and contractility. The potassium level should be carefully followed in patients with uremia, Addison's disease, vomiting and diarrhea, and steroid therapy and in patients taking potassium-depleting diuretics. K must be closely monitored in patients taking digitalis-like drugs because cardiac arrhythmias may be induced by hypokalemia and digoxin.

Interfering factors

- Hemolysis of blood during venipuncture causes increased levels.
- Drugs that may cause *decreased* levels include amphotericin B, diuretics (potassium wasting), glucose infusions, insulin, laxatives, lithium carbonate, and sodium polystyrene sulfonate (Kayexalate).

Procedure and patient care

Before

- Tell the patient that no special diet or fasting is required.

During
- Collect approximately 5 to 7 ml of venous blood in a red- or green-top tube.
- Avoid hemolysis.

After
- Apply pressure to the venipuncture site.

Abnormal findings

▲ **Increased levels (hyperkalemia)**
Excessive dietary intake
Excessive IV intake
Acute or chronic renal failure
Hypoaldosteronism
Aldosterone-inhibiting diuretics
Crush injury to tissues
Hemolysis
Transfusion of hemolyzed blood
Infection
Acidosis
Dehydration

▼ **Decreased levels (hypokalemia)**
Deficient dietary intake
Deficient IV intake
Burns
Gastrointestinal disorders (e.g., diarrhea, vomiting)
Diuretics
Hyperaldosteronism
Cushing's syndrome
Renal tubular acidosis
Licorice ingestion
Insulin administration
Glucose administration
Ascites
Renal artery stenosis
Cystic fibrosis
Trauma
Surgery

P

notes

prealbumin (PAB, Thyroxine-binding prealbumin [TBPA], Thyretin, Transthyretin)

Type of test Blood; urine (24-hour); cerebrospinal fluid (CSF) analysis

Normal findings

Serum
Adult/elderly: 15-36 mg/dl or 150-360 mg/L (SI units)
Child
   Cord: 13 mg/dl or 130 mg/L (SI units)
   1 year: 10 mg/dl or 100 mg/L
   2-36 months: 16-28 mg/dl or 160-280 mg/L

Possible critical values Serum prealbumin levels <10.7 mg/dl indicate severe nutritional deficiency.

Test explanation

Prealbumin is one of the major plasma proteins. Since prealbumin levels in serum fluctuate more rapidly in response to alterations in synthetic rate than do those of other serum proteins, clinical interest in the quantification of serum prealbumin has centered on its usefulness as a marker of nutritional status. Its half-life of 1.9 days is much less than the 21-day half-life of albumin. Because prealbumin has a short half-life, it is a sensitive indicator of any change affecting protein synthesis and catabolism. Because of this, prealbumin is frequently ordered to monitor the effectiveness of total parenteral nutrition (TPN).

Prealbumin is significantly reduced in hepatobiliary disease because of impaired synthesis. Prealbumin is also a negative acute-phase reactant protein; serum levels decrease in inflammation, malignancy, and protein-wasting diseases of the intestines or kidneys. Since zinc is required for synthesis of prealbumin, low levels occur with a zinc deficiency. Increased levels of prealbumin occur in Hodgkin's disease and during chronic kidney disease.

Procedure and patient care

Before
- Tell the patient that no food or fluid restrictions are needed.

During
- Collect a venous blood sample in a red-top tube.

After
- Apply pressure to the venipuncture site.

Abnormal findings

▲ **Increased levels**
Some cases of nephrotic
  syndrome
Hodgkin's disease
Chronic kidney disease
Pregnancy

▼ **Decreased levels**
Malnutrition
Liver damage
Burns
Salicylate poisoning
Inflammation

notes

- Urine pregnancy tests can vary according to the dilution of the urine. HCH levels may not be detectable in dilute urine but may be quite detectable in concentrated urine.

Procedure and patient care

Before

- If a urine specimen will be collected, give the patient a urine container the evening before so that she can provide a first-voided morning specimen. This specimen generally contains the greatest concentration of HCG.

During

- Collect the first-voided urine specimen for urine testing.
- Collect approximately 7 to 10 ml of venous blood in a red-top tube for serum testing. Avoid hemolysis.

After

- Apply pressure to the venipuncture site.
- Emphasize to the patient the importance of antepartal health care.

Abnormal findings

▲ **Increased levels**
Pregnancy
Ectopic pregnancy
Hydatidiform mole of the uterus
Choriocarcinoma of the uterus, testes, or ovaries
Tumor

▼ **Decreased levels**
Threatened abortion
Incomplete abortion
Dead fetus

notes

Type of test Blood

Normal findings

Adult/elderly
Total protein: 6.4-8.3 g/dl or 64-83 g/L (SI units)
Albumin: 3.5-5 g/dl or 35-50 g/L (SI units)
Globulin: 2.3-3.4 g/dl
  Alpha$_1$ globulin: 0.1-0.3 g/dl or 1-3 g/L (SI units)
  Alpha$_2$ globulin: 0.6-1 g/dl or 6-10 g/L (SI units)
  Beta globulin: 0.7-1.1 g/dl or 7-11 g/L (SI units)
Children
  Total protein
    Premature infant: 4.2-7.6 g/dl
    Newborn: 4.6-7.4 g/dl
    Infant: 6-6.7 g/dl
    Child: 6.2-8 g/dl
  Albumin
    Premature infant: 3-4.2 g/dl
    Newborn: 3.5-5.4 g/dl
    Infant: 4.4-5.4 g/dl
    Child: 4-5.9 g/dl

P

Test explanation

Albumin and globulin constitute most of the protein within the body and are measured in the total protein. *Albumin* is a protein that is formed within the liver. It makes up approximately 60% of the total protein. Albumin is synthesized within the liver and is therefore a measure of hepatic function. When disease affects the liver cell, the serum albumin level is greatly decreased. Because the half-life of albumin is 12 to 18 days, however, severe impairment of hepatic albumin synthesis may not be recognized until after that period.

Alpha$_1$ globulins are mostly alpha$_1$ antitrypsin. Some transporting proteins such as thyroid and cortisol-binding globulin also contribute to this electrophoretic zone. Alpha$_2$ globulins include serum haptoglobins (bind hemoglobin during hemolysis), ceruloplasmin (carrier for copper), prothrombin, and cholinesterase (an enzyme used in the catabolism of acetylcholine). Beta globulins include lipoproteins, transferrin, plasminogen, and complement proteins; beta$_2$ globulins include fibrinogen. Gamma globulins are the immune globulins (antibodies) (see p. 162).

Serum albumin and globulin are measures of nutrition. Malnourished patients, especially after surgery, have a greatly decreased level of serum proteins. Burn patients and patients who have protein-losing enteropathies and nephropathies have low levels of protein, despite normal synthesis. Pregnancy, especially the third trimester, is usually associated with reduced total proteins.

Serum protein electrophoresis can separate the various components of blood protein into bands or zones according to their electrical charge. Several well-established electrophoretic patterns have been identified and can be associated with specific diseases (Table 2).

Procedure and patient care

Before
- Tell the patient that no fasting is usually required.

During
- Collect approximately 5 to 7 ml of blood in a red-top tube.

After
- Apply pressure to the venipuncture site. Patients with liver dysfunction often have prolonged clotting times.

Abnormal findings

▲ Increased albumin levels
Dehydration

▼ Decreased albumin levels
Malnutrition
Pregnancy
Liver disease
Protein-losing enteropathies
Protein-losing nephropathies
Third-space losses
Overhydration
Increased capillary permeability
Inflammatory disease
Familial idiopathic dysproteinemia

TABLE 2 Protein electrophoresis patterns in specific diseases

Pattern	Electrophoresis	Disease
Acute reaction	↓ Albumin ↑ Alpha$_2$ globulin	Acute infections, tissue necrosis, burns, surgery, stress, myocardial infarction
Chronic inflammatory	sl. ↓ Albumin sl. ↑ Gamma globulin $\overline{N}$ Alpha$_2$ globulin	Chronic infection, granulomatous diseases, cirrhosis, rheumatoid-collagen diseases
Nephrotic syndrome	↓↓ Albumin ↑↑ Alpha$_2$-globulin $\overline{N}$↑ Beta globulin	Nephrotic syndrome
Far-advanced cirrhosis	↓ Albumin ↑ Gamma globulin Incorporation of beta and gamma peaks	Far-advanced cirrhosis
Polyclonal gamma globulin elevation	↑↑ Gamma globulin with a broad peak	Cirrhosis, chronic infection, sarcoidosis, tuberculosis, endocarditis, rheumatoid-collagen disease
Hypogamma-globulinemia	↓ Gamma globulin with normal other globulin levels	Light-chain multiple myeloma
Monoclonal gammopathy	Thin spikes in gamma globulin	Myeloma, macroglobulinemia, gammopathies

↓, Decreased; ↑, increased; sl. ↓, slightly decreased; sl. ↑, slightly increased; $\overline{N}$ normal; ↓↓, greatly decreased; ↑↑, greatly increased.

pulmonary stress testing can also be performed to provide data concerning the patient's pulmonary reserve.

Spirometry is performed first. On the basis of age, height, weight, race, and sex, normal values for the volumes and flow rates can be predicted. If the actual values are greater than 80% of predicted values, the person is considered normal. Spirometry provides information about obstruction or restriction of air flow. If airflow rates are significantly diminished (<60% of normal), spirometry can be repeated after bronchodilators are administered by nebulizer. If airflow rates are improved by 20%, the chronic use of bronchodilators may be recommended to the patient. Measurement of lung capacities (combination of two or more lung volumes) can be performed.

Gas exchange studies measure the diffusing capacity of the lung (D_L) (i.e., the amount of gas exchanged across the alveolar-capillary membrane per minute). Arterial blood gases (see p. 21) are also a part of pulmonary function studies as the information obtained is used in calculations of lung function data.

PFTs routinely include determination of the following:

Forced vital capacity. FVC is the amount of air that can be forcefully expelled from a maximally inflated lung position.

Forced expiratory volume in 1 second. FEV_1 is the volume of air expelled during the first second of the FVC.

Maximal midexpiratory flow. MMEF is the maximal rate of airflow through the pulmonary tree during forced expiration. This is also called *forced midexpiratory flow.*

Maximal volume ventilation. MVV, formerly called *maximal breathing capacity,* is the maximal volume of air that the patient can breathe in and out during 1 minute.

Tidal volume. TV or V_T is the volume of air inspired and expired with each normal respiration.

Inspiratory reserve volume. IRV is the maximal volume of air that can be inspired from the end of a normal inspiration.

Expiratory reserve volume. ERV is the maximal volume of air that can be exhaled after a normal expiration.

Residual volume. RV is the volume of air remaining in the lungs following forced expiration.

Inspiratory capacity. IC is the maximal amount of air that can be inspired after a normal expiration (IC = TV + IRV).

Functional residual volume. FRV is the amount of air left in the lungs after a normal expiration (FRV = ERV + RV).

Vital capacity. VC is the maximal amount of air that can be expired after a maximal inspiration (VC = TV + IRV + ERV).

Total lung capacity. TLC is the volume to which the lungs can be expanded with the greatest inspiratory effort (TLC = TV + IRV + ERV + RV).

Minute volume. MV, sometimes called *minute ventilation,* is the volume of air inhaled and exhaled per minute.

Dead space. Dead space is the part of the tidal volume that does not participate in alveolar gas exchange. This would include the air within the trachea.

Forced expiratory flow$_{200-1200}$. $FEF_{200-1200}$ is the airflow rate of expired air between 200 ml and 1200 ml during the FVC.

Forced expiratory flow$_{25-75}$. FEF_{25-75} is the airflow rate of expired air between 25% and 75% of the flow during the FVC.

Peak inspiratory flow rate. PIFR is the flow rate of inspired air during maximum inspiration.

Procedure and patient care

Before

- Inform the patient that cooperation is necessary to obtain accurate results.
- Instruct the patient not to use bronchodilators or smoke for 6 hours before this test (if requested by physician).
- Withhold the use of small-dose meter inhalers and aerosol therapy before this study.
- Measure and record the patient's height and weight before this study to determine the predicted values.

During

- Note the following procedural steps:

Spirometry and airflow rates
1. The patient breathes through a sterile mouthpiece and into a spirometer to measure and record the desired values.
2. The patient is asked to inhale as deeply as possible and then forcibly exhale as much air as possible. This is repeated several times.
3. The patient is asked to breathe in and out as deeply and frequently as possible for 15 seconds. The total volume breathed is recorded and multiplied by 4 to obtain the MVV.

P

4. The patient is asked to breathe in and out normally into the spirometer and then exhale forcibly from the end tidal volume expiration point. This provides measurement of ERV.

5. The patient is asked to breathe in and out normally into the spirometer and then inhale forcibly from the end tidal volume expiration point. This provides measurement of IC.

6. The patient is asked to breathe in and out maximally (but not forced). This is a measure of VC and the calculated TLC.

Gas exchange/diffusing capacity of the lung (D_L)

1. The D_L of CO is usually measured by having the patient inhale a CO mixture.

After

- Note that patients with severe respiratory problems are occasionally exhausted after the testing and will need rest.

Abnormal findings

Pulmonary fibrosis
Interstitial lung diseases
Tumor
Chest wall trauma
Emphysema
Chronic bronchitis
Asthma
Inhalant pneumonitis
Post-pneumonectomy
Bronchiectasis
Airway infection
Pneumonia
Neuromuscular disease
Hypersensitivity bronchospasm

notes

red blood cell count (RBC count, Erythrocyte count)

Type of test Blood

Normal findings (million/mm^3 or million/μl)

Adult/elderly
  Male: 4.7-6.1
  Female: 4.2-5.4
Children
  Newborn: 4.8-7.1
  2-8 wks: 4-6
  2-6 mos: 3.5-5.5
  6 mos-1 yr: 3.5-5.2
  1-6 yr: 4-5.5
  6-18 yr: 4-5.5

Test explanation

  This test is a count of the number of circulating red blood cells (RBCs) in 1 mm^3 of peripheral venous blood. The RBC is routinely performed as part of a complete blood count.

  When the value is decreased by more than 10% of the expected normal value, the patient is said to be anemic. Low RBC values are caused by many factors, including the following:

  1. Hemorrhage, as in gastrointestinal bleeding or trauma
  2. Hemolysis, as in glucose-6-phosphate dehydrogenase deficiency, spherocytosis, or secondary splenomegaly
  3. Dietary deficiency, as of iron or vitamin B$_{12}$
  4. Genetic aberrations, as in sickle cell anemia or thalassemia
  5. Drug ingestion, as of chloramphenicol, hydantoins, or quinidine
  6. Marrow failure, as in fibrosis, leukemia, or antineoplastic chemotherapy
  7. Chronic illness, as in tumor or sepsis
  8. Other organ failure, as in renal disease

RBC counts greater than normal can be physiologically induced as a result of the body's requirements for greater oxygen-carrying capacity (e.g., at high altitudes). Diseases that produce chronic hypoxia (e.g., congenital heart disease) also provoke this physiologic increase in RBCs. Polycythemia vera is a neoplastic condition involving uncontrolled production of RBCs.

R

Interfering factors

- Hydration status: Dehydration factitiously increases the RBC count, and overhydration decreases the RBC count.

Procedure and patient care

Before

- Tell the patient that no fasting is required.

During

- Collect approximately 5 to 7 ml of blood in a lavender-top tube.
- Thoroughly mix the blood with the anticoagulant by tilting the tube.
- Avoid hemolysis.

After

- Apply pressure to the venipuncture site.

Abnormal findings

▲ Increased levels	▼ Decreased levels
High altitude	Hemorrhage
Congenital heart disease	Hemolysis
Polycythemia vera	Anemia
Dehydration/ hemoconcentration	Hemoglobinopathy
Cor pulmonale	Advanced cancer
Pulmonary fibrosis	Bone marrow fibrosis
	Leukemia
	Antineoplastic chemo- therapy
	Chronic illness
	Renal failure
	Overhydration
	Multiple myeloma
	Pernicious anemia
	Rheumatoid disease
	Subacute endocarditis
	Pregnancy
	Dietary deficiency

notes

renal scanning (Kidney scan, Radiorenography, Renography, Radionuclide renal imaging, Nuclear imaging of the kidney, DMSA renal scan, DTPA renal scan, Captopril renal scan)

Type of test Nuclear scan

Normal findings Normal size, shape, and function of the kidney

Test explanation

Renal scans are to indicate the perfusion, function, and structure of the kidneys. They are also used to indicate the presence of ureteral obstruction or renovascular hypertension. Because this study uses no iodinated dyes (except when iodohippurate is used), it is safe to use on patients who have iodine allergies or compromised renal function. Renal scans are used to monitor renal function in patients with known renal disease. This scan also plays a large part in the diagnosis of renal transplant rejection.

There are several different kinds of renal scans, depending on what information is needed to be obtained. Different isotopes may be more suitable for different scans, based on the manner in which the kidney handles the radioisotope.

Renal blood flow (perfusion) scan

This type of renal scan is used to evaluate the blood flow to each kidney. It is used to identify renal artery stenosis, renovascular hypertension, and rejection of renal transplant. Also, it is used to demonstrate hypervascular lesions (renal cell carcinoma) in the kidney.

Decreased gamma activity is noted in the kidney with arterial stenosis or renovascular hypertension. Decreased activity relative to the aorta is noted in a transplanted kidney that is experiencing rejection. Localized increased gamma activity is noted in the kidney that contains a hypervascular tumor (cancer).

Renal structural scan

This type of renal scan is performed to outline the structure of the kidney to identify pathology that may alter normal anatomic structure (e.g., tumor, cyst, abscess). Congenital disorders (e.g., hypoplasia or aplasia of the kidney, malposition of the kidney) can also be detected. A filling defect in the renal parenchyma may indicate a tumor, cyst, abscess, or infarction. Horseshoe-shaped

R

kidney, pelvic kidney, or absence of a kidney may be evident. Also, information concerning postrenal transplants can be obtained with this scan. Anatomic alterations in the parenchymal distribution of tracer may indicate transplant rejection. Tc-DTPA or DSMA can be used for this scan.

Renal function scan (renogram)

Renal function can be determined by documenting the capability of the kidney to take up and excrete a particular radioisotope. A well-functioning kidney can be expected to rapidly assimilate the isotope and then excrete it. A poorly functioning kidney will not be able to take up the isotope rapidly nor excrete it in a timely manner. Renal function can be monitored by serially repeating this test and comparing results.

Renal hypertension scan

This scan is used to identify the presence and location of renovascular hypertension.

Renal obstruction scan

This scan is performed to identify obstruction of the outflow tract of the kidney caused by obstruction of the renal pelvis, ureter, or bladder outlet.

Often several of these scans are combined to obtain the maximum information about the renal system as possible. A *triple renal study* may use all of these techniques to evaluate renal blood perfusion, structure, and excretion.

Contraindications

- Patients who are pregnant because of the risk of fetal damage

Procedure and patient care

Before

- Do not schedule a renal scan within 24 hours after an intravenous pyelogram.
- Note that Lugol's solution (10 drops) may be ordered if ^{131}I orthoiodohippurate is used. This minimizes thyroid uptake of the radioisotope.
- Remind the patient to void before the scan.
- Tell the patient that no sedation or fasting is required but that good hydration is essential.
- Instruct the patient to drink two to three glasses of water before the scan.

During

- Note the following procedural steps:
    1. A peripheral IV injection of radionuclide is given. It takes only minutes for the radioisotopes to be concentrated in the kidneys.
    2. While the patient assumes a prone or sitting position, a gamma ray scintography camera is passed over the kidney area and records the radioactive uptake on film.
    3. Unique features of the various scans:
        a. For a *Lasix renal scan* or a *diuretic renal scan,* images are obtained for 10 to 20 minutes; then 40 mg of Lasix is administered IV, and another 20 minutes of images are obtained.
        b. For the *captopril renal scan,* the patient is scanned after the administration of captopril.
        c. For the *renal blood flow* and the *renal function scans,* scanning is started immediately after the injection
        d. For *structural renal scans,* the patient is asked to lie still for the entire time of the scan (30 minutes).

After

- Tell the patient that the radioactive substance is usually excreted from the body within 6 to 24 hours. Encourage the patient to drink fluids.

Abnormal findings

Urinary obstruction
Pyelonephritis
Renovascular hypertension
Absence of kidney function
Renal infarction
Renal arterial atherosclerosis
Glomerulonephritis
Renal tumor
Congenital abnormalities
Renal trauma
Transplant rejection
Acute tubular necrosis
Renal abscess
Renal cyst

R

reticulocyte count (Retic count)

Type of test Blood

Normal findings

Reticulocyte count:
   Adult/elderly/child: 0.5% to 2%
   Infant: 0.5% to 3.1%
   Newborn: 2.5% to 6.5%
Reticulocyte index: 1.0

Test explanation

The reticulocyte count is a test for determining bone marrow function and evaluating erythropoietic activity. This test is also useful in classifying anemias. A reticulocyte is an immature red blood cell (RBC) that can be readily identified under a microscope. Normally there are a small number of reticulocytes in the bloodstream.

The reticulocyte count gives an indication of RBC production by the bone marrow. Increased reticulocyte counts indicate that the marrow is putting an increased number of RBCs into the bloodstream, usually in response to anemia. A normal or low reticulocyte count in a patient with anemia indicates that the marrow response to the anemia by way of production of RBCs is inadequate and is perhaps contributing to or is the cause of the anemia (as in aplastic anemia, iron deficiency, vitamin B_{12} deficiency, or depletion of iron stores). An elevated reticulocyte count found in patients with a normal hemogram indicates increased RBC production compensating for an ongoing loss of RBCs (hemolysis or hemorrhage).

To determine if a reticulocyte count indicates an appropriate erythropoietic (RBC marrow) response in patients with anemia and a decreased hematocrit, one should calculate the *reticulocyte index:*

Reticulocyte index =

$$\text{Reticulocyte count (in \%)} \times \frac{\text{Patient's hematocrit}}{\text{Normal hematocrit}}$$

The reticulocyte index in a patient with a good marrow response to the anemia should be 1.0. If it is below 1.0, even though the reticulocyte count is elevated, the bone marrow response is inadequate in its ability to compensate.

Procedure and patient care

Before
- Tell the patient that no fasting is required.

During
- Collect approximately 5 to 7 ml of venous blood in a lavender-top tube.

After
- Apply pressure to the venipuncture site.

Abbnormal findings

▲ **Increased levels**
Hemolytic anemia
Sickle cell anemia
Hemorrhage (3 to 4 days later)
Postsplenectomy
Erythroblastosis fetalis
Pregnancy
Leukemias
Recovery from nutritional anemias

▼ **Decreased levels**
Pernicious anemia
Folic acid deficiency
Adrenocortical hypofunction
Aplastic anemia
Radiation therapy
Marrow failure
Anterior pituitary hypofunction
Chronic infection
Cirrhosis
Malignancy

notes

rubella antibody test (German measles test, Hemagglutination inhibition [HAI])

Type of test Blood

Normal findings

Method	Result	Interpretation
HAI titer	<1:8	No immunity to rubella
HAI titer	>1:20	Immune to rubella
LA	Negative	No immunity to rubella
ELISA—IgM	<0.9 IU/ml	No infection
ELISA—IgM	>1.1 IU/ml	Active infection
ELISA—IgG	<7 IU/ml	No immunity to rubella
ELISA—IgG	>10 IU/ml	Immune to rubella

LA, Latex agglutination; *ELISA*, enzyme-linked immunosorbent assay.

Possible critical values Evidence of susceptibility in pregnant women with recent exposure to rubella

Test explanation

Screening for rubella antibodies is done to detect immunity to rubella. These tests detect the presence of IgG and/or IgM antibodies to rubella (the causative agent for German measles). They become elevated a few days to a few weeks after the onset of the rash, depending on what method of testing is used. IgM tends to disappear after about 6 weeks. IgG, however, persists at low but detectable levels for years. The term TORCH (toxoplasmosis, other, rubella, cytomegalovirus, herpes) has been applied to infections with recognized detrimental effects on the fetus.

Anti-rubella antibody testing is also used to diagnose rubella in infants (congenital rubella). IgM anti-rubella antibodies cannot pass through the placenta. If an infant has IgM antibodies, acute congenital or newborn rubella is suspected. Antibody testing is often used in children with congenital abnormalities which may have come from congenital rubella infection.

Procedure and patient care

Before

- Explain the purpose of the test to the patient.

During

- Collect approximately 7 ml of venous blood in a red-top tube.

After

- Apply pressure to the venipuncture site.
- Inform the patient when to return for a follow-up HAI titer, if indicated.

Abnormal findings

Active rubella infection
Previous rubella infection leading to immunity

notes

R

semen analysis (Sperm count, Sperm examination, Seminal cytology, Semen examination)

Type of test Fluid analysis

Normal findings

Volume: 2-5 ml
Liquefaction time: 20 to 30 minutes after collection
pH: 7.12-8.00
Sperm count (density): 50-200 million/ml
Sperm motility: 60% to 80% actively motile
Sperm morphology: 70% to 90% normally shaped

Test explanation

Semen analysis is one of the most important aspects of the fertility workup because the cause of a woman's inability to conceive often lies with the man. Sperm is examined for volume, sperm count, motility, and morphology.

The freshly collected semen is first measured for volume. After liquefaction of the white, gelatinous ejaculate, a sperm count is done. Men with very low or very high counts likely are infertile. The motility of the sperm is then evaluated. Morphology is studied by staining a semen preparation and calculating the number of normal versus abnormal sperm forms.

Semen production depends on the function of the testicles. Semen analysis is a measure of testicular function. Inadequate sperm production can be the result of primary gonadal failure (Klinefelter syndrome, infection, radiation, or surgical orchidectomy) or secondary gonadal failure (caused by pituitary diseases). Men with *aspermia* (no sperm) or *oligospermia* (20 million/ml) should be evaluated endocrinologically for pituitary, thyroid, or testicular aberrations.

In addition to its value in infertility workups, semen analysis is also helpful in documenting adequate sterilization after a vasectomy. It is usually performed 6 weeks after the surgery. If any sperm are seen, the adequacy of the vasectomy must be questioned.

Procedure and patient care

Before

- Instruct the patient to abstain from sexual activity for 2 to 3 days before collecting the specimen.

- Give the patient the proper container for the sperm collection.
- For evaluation of the adequacy of vasectomy, the patient should ejaculate once or twice before the day of examination.

During

- Note that semen is best collected by ejaculation into a clean container. For best results, the specimen should be collected in the physician's office or laboratory by masturbation.
- Note that less satisfactory specimens can be obtained in the patient's home by coitus interruptus or masturbation. Note the following procedural steps:
  1. Instruct the patient to deliver these home specimens to the laboratory within 1 hour after collection.
  2. Tell the patient to avoid excessive heat and cold during transportation of the specimen.

After

- Record the date of the previous semen emission, along with the collection time and date of the fresh specimen.

Abnormal findings

Infertility
Vasectomy (obstruction of vas deferens)
Orchitis
Testicular atrophy
Testicular failure
Hyperpyrexia

S

notes

sodium, blood (Na⁺)

Type of test Blood

Normal findings

Adult/elderly: 136-145 mEq/L or 136/145 mmol/L (SI units)
Child: 136-145 mEq/L
Infant: 134-150 mEq/L
Newborn: 134-144 mEq/L

Possible critical values <120 or >160 mEq/L

Test explanation

Sodium is the major cation in the extracellular space. Physiologically water and sodium are very closely interrelated. As free body water is increased, serum sodium is diluted, and the concentration may decrease. If free body water were to decrease, the serum sodium concentration would rise.

An average dietary intake of approximately 90 to 250 mEq/day is needed to maintain sodium balance in adults. Symptoms of hyponatremia may include weakness, confusion, lethargy, stupor, and coma. Symptoms of hypernatremia include dry mucous membranes, thirst, agitation, restlessness, hyperreflexia, mania, and convulsions.

Procedure and patient care

Before

- Tell the patient that no food or fluid is restricted.

During

- Collect 5 to 10 ml of venous blood in a red- or green-top tube.
- If the patient is receiving an IV infusion, obtain blood from the opposite arm.

After

- Apply pressure to the venipuncture site.

Abnormal findings

▲ **Increased levels (hypernatremia)**

Increased sodium intake
Excessive dietary intake
Excessive sodium in IV fluids

Decreased sodium loss
Cushing's syndrome
Hyperaldosteronism

Excessive free body water loss
Excessive sweating
Extensive thermal burns
Diabetes insipidus
Osmotic diuresis

▼ **Decreased levels (hyponatremia)**

Decreased sodium intake
Deficient dietary intake
Deficient sodium in IV fluids

Increased sodium loss
Addison's disease
Diarrhea
Vomiting or nasogastric aspiration
Diuretic administration
Chronic renal insufficiency

Increased free body water
Excessive oral water intake
Excessive IV water intake
Congestive heart failure
Syndrome of inappropriate secretion of ADH (SIADH)
Osmotic dilution

Third-space losses of sodium
Ascites
Peripheral edema
Pleural effusion
Intraluminal bowel loss (ileus or mechanical obstruction)

S

notes

stool for occult blood (Stool for OB)

Type of test Stool

Normal findings No occult blood within stool

Test explanation

Benign and malignant GI tumors, ulcers, inflammatory bowel disease, arteriovenous malformations, diverticulosis, and hematobilia (hemobilia) can cause OB within the stool. Other more common abnormalities (e.g., hemorrhoids, swallowed blood from oral or nasal pharyngeal bleeding) may also cause OB within the stool. This test can detect occult blood when as little as 5 ml of blood is lost per day.

This test is a part of every routine physical examination. It is also a part of routine screening of asymptomatic individuals over the age of 50 years.

Interfering factors

- Vigorous exercise
- Bleeding gums following a dental procedure
- Ingestion of red meat within 3 days before testing
- Ingestion of fish, turnips, and horseradish
- Drugs that may cause GI bleeding include anticoagulants, aspirin, colchicine, iron preparations (large doses), nonsteroidal antiarthritics, and steroids

Procedure and patient care

Before

- Instruct the patient to refrain from eating any red meat for at least 3 days before the test.
- Instruct the patient as to the method of obtaining appropriate stool specimens. Many procedures are available (e.g., specimen cards, tissue wipes, test paper). Tests may be done at home with specimen cards (Hemoccult) and mailed when collected.
- Inform the patient as to the need for multiple specimens obtained on separate days to increase the test's accuracy.
- Note that in some centers a high-residue diet is recommended to increase the abrasive effect of the stool.
- Be gentle in obtaining stool by digital rectal examination. Traumatic digital examination can cause a false-positive

stool, especially in patients with prior anorectal disease such as hemorrhoids.

During

Hemoccult slide test

- Place a stool sample on one side of guaiac paper.
- Place two drops of developer on the other side.
- Note that a bluish discoloration indicates OB in the stool.

Tablet test

- Place a stool sample on the developer paper.
- Place a tablet on top of the stool specimen.
- Put two or three drops of tap water on the tablet and allow to flow onto the paper.
- Note that a bluish discoloration indicates OB in the stool.

After

- If the tests are positive, inquire whether the patient violated any of the preparation recommendations.

Abnormal findings

GI tumor
Polyps
Ulcer
Varices
Inflammatory bowel disease
Diverticulosis
Ischemic bowel disease
GI trauma
Recent GI surgery
Hemorrhoids
Esophagitis
Gastritis

S

notes

therapeutic drug monitoring (TDM)

Type of test Blood

Normal findings See Table 3.

Test explanation

Therapeutic drug monitoring (TDM) entails taking measurements of blood drug levels to determine effective drug dosages and to prevent toxicity. It is also used to identify noncompliant patients. Patient age and size, extent and rate of drug absorption or excretion, and metabolic rate can all affect drug levels. Measurement of drug levels is very important in patients who are beyond the normal range in regard to variables that affect drug metabolism. TDM is helpful in patients who take other medicines that may affect drug levels or act in a synergistic or antagonistic manner with the drug to be tested. TDM is helpful in prescribing medicines (e.g., antiarrhythmics, bronchodilators, antibiotics, anticonvulsants, cardiotonics) that have a very narrow therapeutic margin (i.e., the difference between therapeutic and toxic drug levels is small).

Table 3 lists the therapeutic and toxic ranges for most patients. These ranges may not apply to all patients because clinical response is influenced by many factors (e.g., noncompliance, concurrent drug use, other clinical conditions, patient's age and size, extent and rate of drug absorption, metabolism). Also, note that different laboratories use different units for reporting test results and normal ranges. It is important that sufficient time pass between the administration of the medication and the collection of the blood sample to allow for therapeutic levels to occur.

Blood samples can be taken at the drug's *peak* level (the highest concentration) or at the *trough* level (the lowest concentration). Peak levels are useful when testing for toxicity, and trough levels are useful for demonstrating a satisfactory therapeutic level. Trough levels are often referred to as *residual* levels. The time when the sample should be drawn after the last dose of the medication varies according to whether a peak or trough level is requested and according to the half-life of the drug.

Procedure and patient care

Before

- Tell the patient that no food or fluid restrictions are needed.

TABLE 3 Therapeutic drug monitoring data

Drug	Use	Therapeutic level*	Toxic level*
Acetaminophen	Analgesic, antipyretic	Depends on use	>250 μg/ml
Amikacin	Antibiotic	15-25 μg/ml	>25 μg/ml
Aminophylline	Bronchodilator	10-20 μg/ml	>20 μg/ml
Amitriptyline	Antidepressant	120-150 ng/ml	>500 ng/ml
Carbamazepine	Anticonvulsant	5-12 μg/ml	>12 μg/ml
Chloramphenicol	Antiinfective	10-20 μg/ml	>25 μg/ml
Desipramine	Antidepressant	150-300 ng/ml	>500 ng/ml
Digitoxin	Cardiac glycoside	15-25 ng/ml	>25 ng/ml
Digoxin	Cardiac glycoside	0.8-2.0 ng/ml	>2.4 ng/ml
Disopyramide	Antiarrhythmic	2-5 μg/ml	>5 μg/ml
Ethosuximide	Anticonvulsant	40-100 μg/ml	>100 μg/ml
Gentamicin	Antibiotic	5-10 μg/ml	>12 μg/ml
Imipramine	Antidepressant	150-300 ng/ml	>500 ng/ml
Kanamycin	Antibiotic	20-25 μg/ml	>35 μg/ml
Lidocaine	Antiarrhythmic	1.5-5.0 μg/ml	>5 μg/ml

Continued

*Levels vary according to the institution performing the test.

T

TABLE 3 Therapeutic drug monitoring data—cont'd

Drug	Use	Therapeutic level*	Toxic level*
Lithium	Manic episodes of manic-depression psychosis	0.8-1.2 mEq/L	>2.0 mEq/L
Methotrexate	Antitumor agent	>0.01 μmol	>10 μmol/24 hr
Nortriptyline	Antidepressant	50-150 ng/ml	>500 ng/ml
Phenobarbital	Anticonvulsant	10-30 μg/ml	>40 μg/ml
Phenytoin	Anticonvulsant	10-20 μg/ml	>30 μg/ml
Primidone	Anticonvulsant	5-12 μg/ml	>15 μg/ml
Procainamide	Antiarrhythmic	4-10 μg/ml	>16 μg/ml
Propranolol	Antiarrhythmic	50-100 ng/ml	>150 ng/ml
Quinidine	Antiarrhythmic	2-5 μg/ml	>10 μg/ml
Salicylate	Antipyretic, antiinflammatory, analgesic	100-250 μg/ml	>300 μg/ml
Theophylline	Bronchodilator	10-20 μg/ml	>20 μg/ml
Tobramycin	Antibiotic	5-10 μg/ml	>12 μg/ml
Valproic acid	Anticonvulsant	50-100 μg/ml	>100 μg/ml

During

- Collect approximately 7 to 10 ml of venous blood in a tube designated by the laboratory. *Peak* levels are usually obtained 1 to 2 hours after oral intake, approximately 1 hour after IM administration, and approximately 30 minutes after IV administration. *Residual* (trough) levels are usually obtained shortly before (0 to 15 minutes) the next scheduled dose. Consult with the pharmacy for specific times.

After

- Clearly mark all blood samples with the following information: patient's name, diagnosis, name of drug, time of last drug ingestion, time of sample, and any other medications the patient is currently taking.

Abnormal findings

Nontherapeutic levels of drugs
Toxic levels of drugs

notes

THYROID HORMONE TESTING
thyroxine, total (T4, Thyroxine screen)
thyroxine, free (FT4)
triiodothyronine (T3)

Type of test Blood

Normal findings
T4: 4-12 μg/dl
FT4: 0.8-2.7 ng/dl
T3: 40-180 ng/dl

Possible critical values
T4:
Newborn: <7 μg/dl
Adult: <2 μg/dl if myxedema coma possible; >20 μg/dl if thyroid storm possible

Test explanation

The serum thyroxine (T4) study is a direct measurement of the total amount of T4 present in the patient's blood. T4 makes up nearly all of what we call thyroid hormone. Greater-than-normal levels indicate hyperthyroid states, and subnormal values are seen in hypothyroid states. Newborns are screened by T4 tests to detect hypothyroidism. This is a very reliable test of thyroid function. T4 testing is also used to monitor replacement and suppressive therapy.

Because T4 is bound by serum proteins such as TBG, any increase in these proteins (as in pregnant women and patients taking oral contraceptives) will cause factitiously elevated levels of T4 and, to some extent, triiodothyronine (T3). FT4 is used to determine thyroid function when the patient has concurrent clinical situations that may alter protein blood levels. Only 1% to 5% of total T4 is unbound or "free." The free T4 is the metabolically active thyroid hormone. When measuring total T4, the bound and the unbound are measured.

Serum T3 test is another accurate measure of thyroid function. T3 is less stable than T4 and occurs in minute quantities. Only about 7% to 10% of thyroid hormone is composed of T3. Seventy percent of that T3 is bound to proteins (thyroid-binding globulin [TBG] and albumen). This test is a measurement of total T3, (i.e., the free and the bound T3). Generally, when the T3 level is below normal, the patient is in a hypothyroid state.

Other severe nonthyroidal diseases can decrease T3 levels by diminishing the conversion of T4 to T3 in the liver. This makes T3 levels less useful in indicating hypothyroid states. Because of this, T3 levels are mostly just used to assist in the diagnosis of hyperthyroid states. An elevated T3 indicates hyperthyroidism, especially when the T4 is also elevated. There is a rare form of hyperthyroidism called *T3* toxicosis, in which the T4 is normal and the T3 is elevated.

Interfering factors

- Neonates have higher levels than do older children and adults.
- Prior use of radioisotopes can alter test results as the method used to determine free T4 levels is radioimmunoassay.
- Exogenously administered thyroxine causes elevated free T4 results.
- T4 levels may be increased after x-ray iodinated contrast studies.

Procedure and patient care

Before

- Determine whether the patient is taking any thyroid medication because this will affect test results.
- Tell the patient that no fasting is required.

During

- Collect a venous blood specimen in a red-top tube.
- List on the laboratory slip any drugs that may affect test results.
- For a newborn total T4:
  1. Perform a heel stick to obtain blood.
  2. Thoroughly saturate the circles on the filter paper with blood.

After

- Apply pressure to the collection site.

Abnormal findings

▲ **Increased levels**
  Graves' disease
  Plummer's disease
  Toxic thyroid adenoma
  Acute thyroiditis
  Factitious hyperthyroid-
    ism
  Struma ovarii
  Pregnancy

▼ **Decreased levels**
  Cretinism
  Surgical ablation
  Myxedema
  Pituitary insufficiency
  Hypothalamic failure
  Iodine insufficiency
  Renal failure
  Cushing's disease
  Protein depletion states

notes

thyroid scanning (Thyroid scintiscan)

Type of test   Nuclear scan

Normal findings
Normal size, shape, position, and function of the thyroid gland
No areas of decreased or increased uptake

Test explanation
   Thyroid scanning allows the size, shape, position, and physiologic function of the thyroid gland to be determined with the use of radionuclear scanning. Thyroid nodules are easily detected by this technique. Nodules are classified as functioning (warm/hot) or nonfunctioning (cold), depending on the amount of radionuclide taken up by the nodule. A functioning nodule could represent a benign adenoma or a localized toxic goiter. A nonfunctioning nodule may represent a cyst, carcinoma, nonfunctioning adenoma or goiter, lymphoma, or localized area of thyroiditis.
   Scanning is useful in:
1. Patients with a neck or substernal mass
2. Patients with a thyroid nodule. Thyroid cancers are usually nonfunctioning (cold) nodules.
3. Patients with hyperthyroidism. Scanning assists in differentiating Graves' disease (diffusely enlarged hyperfunctioning thyroid gland) from Plummer's disease (nodular hyperfunctioning gland).
4. Patients with metastatic tumors without a known primary site. A normal scan excludes the thyroid gland as a possible primary site.
5. Patients with a well-differentiated form of thyroid cancer. Areas of metastasis may show up on subsequent whole-body nuclear scans.

Interfering factors
- Iodine-containing foods
- Recent administration of x-ray contrast agents
- Drugs that may affect test results include thyroid drugs

T

Procedure and patient care

Before

- Instruct the patient about medications that need to be restricted for weeks before the test (e.g., thyroid drugs, medications containing iodine).
- Obtain a history concerning previous contrast x-ray studies, nuclear scanning, or intake of any thyroid-suppressive or antithyroid drugs.
- Tell the patient that fasting is usually not required.

During

- Note the following procedural steps:
  1. A standard dose of radioactive technetium is usually given to the patient by mouth. The capsule is tasteless.
  2. Scanning is usually performed 2 hours later.
  3. At the designated time, the patient is placed in a supine position and a detector is passed over the thyroid area.

After

- Assure the patient that the dose of radioactive technetium used in this test is minute and therefore harmless. No isolation and no special urine precautions are needed.

Abnormal findings

Adenoma
Toxic and nontoxic goiter
Cyst
Carcinoma
Lymphoma
Thyroiditis
Graves' disease
Plummer's disease
Metastasis
Hyperthyroidism
Hypothyroidism
Hashimoto's disease

notes

thyroid ultrasound (Thyroid echogram, Thyroid sonogram)

Type of test Ultrasound

Normal findings Normal size, shape, and position of the thyroid gland

Test explanation

Ultrasound examination of the thyroid gland is valuable for distinguishing cystic from solid thyroid nodules. If the nodule is found to be purely cystic (fluid filled), the fluid can simply be aspirated (cysts are not cancerous), and surgery is avoided. If the nodule has a mixed or solid appearance, however, a tumor may be present, and surgery may be required for diagnosis and treatment.

This study may be repeated at intervals to determine the response of a thyroid mass to medical therapy.

Procedure and patient care

Before
- Tell the patient that no fasting or sedation is required.

During
- Note the following procedural steps:
  1. The patient is placed in the supine position with the neck hyperextended.
  2. Gel is applied to the patient's neck.
  3. A sound transducer is passed over the nodule.

After
- Assist the patient in removing the lubricant from his or her neck.

Abnormal findings

Cyst
Tumor
Thyroid adenoma
Thyroid carcinoma
Goiter

T

triglycerides (TGs)

Type of test Blood

Normal findings

Adult/elderly
   Male: 40-160 mg/dl or 0.45-1.81 mmol/L (SI units)
   Female: 35-135 mg/dl or 0.40-1.52 mmol/L (SI units)

Child	Male	Female
0-5 years:	30-86 mg/dl	32-99 mg/dl
6-11 years:	31-108 mg/dl	35-114 mg/dl
12-15 years:	36-138 mg/dl	41-138 mg/dl
16-19 years:	40-163 mg/dl	40-128 mg/dl

Critical values >400 mg/dl

Test explanation

   TGs are a form of fat that exists within the bloodstream. They are transported by very low-density lipoproteins (VLDLs) and low-density lipoproteins (LDLs). TGs are a part of a lipid profile that also evaluates cholesterol (see p. 82) and lipoproteins (see p. 178). A lipid profile is performed to assess the risk of coronary and vascular disease.

Procedure and patient care

Before
- Instruct the patient to fast for 12 to 14 hours before the test. Only water is permitted.
- Tell the patient not to drink alcohol for 24 hours before the test.
- Inform the patient that dietary indiscretion for as much as 2 weeks before this test will influence results.

During
- Collect 5 to 10 ml of venous blood in a red-top tube.

After
- Apply pressure to the venipuncture site.

Abnormal findings

▲ **Increased levels**
Glycogen storage disease
Hyperlipidemias
Hypothyroidism
High-carbohydrate diet
Poorly controlled diabetes
Risk of arteriosclerotic
   occlusive coronary
   disease and peripheral
   vascular disease
Nephrotic syndrome
Hypertension
Alcoholic cirrhosis
Pregnancy
Myocardial infarction

▼ **Decreased levels**
Malabsorption syndrome
Malnutrition
Hyperthyroidism

notes

T

troponins (Cardiac troponin T [cTnT]; Cardiac troponin I [cTnI])

Type of test Blood

Normal findings

Cardiac troponin T <0.2 ng/ml
Cardiac troponin I <0.4 ng/ml

Test explanation

Because of their extraordinary high specificity for myocardial cell injury, cardiac troponin T (cTnT) and cardiac troponin I (cTnI) are very helpful in the evaluation of patients with chest pain. Their use is similar to that of creatine phosphokinase MB (CPK-MB) (see p. 95). Cardiac troponins are more specific for cardiac muscle injury. Cardiac troponins become elevated sooner and remain elevated longer than CPK-MB. This expands the time window of opportunity for diagnosis and thrombolytic treatment of myocardial injury. Finally, cTnT and cTnI are more sensitive to muscle injury than CPK-MB. That is most important in evaluating patients with chest pain.

Cardiac troponins are used in the following cardiac clinical situations:

1. Differentiating cardiac from noncardiac chest pain.
2. Evaluation of patients with unstable angina. If cardiac troponins are elevated, cardiac muscle injury has occurred. Thrombolytic therapy may be indicated because this group of patients is at great risk for a subsequent cardiac event (infarction or sudden death).
3. Detection of reperfusion associated with coronary recanalization. A "wash out" or second peak of cardiac troponin levels accurately indicates reperfusion by way of recanalization or coronary angioplasty.
4. Estimation of myocardial infarction size. Late (4 weeks) cardiac troponin levels are inversely related to left ventricular ejection fraction.
5. Detection of perioperative myocardial infarction.

Interfering factors

- Severe skeletal muscle injury may cause false elevation of cTnT in less than 3% of cases.

Procedure and patient care

Before

- Discuss with the patient the need and reason for frequent venipuncture in diagnosing myocardial infarction.
- Tell the patient that no food or fluid restrictions are necessary.

During

- Collect a venous blood sample in a yellow-top (serum separator) tube. This is usually done initially and 12 hours later followed by daily testing for 3 to 5 days and possibly weekly for 5 to 6 weeks.
- Rotate the venipuncture sites.
- Avoid hemolysis.
- Record the exact time and date of venipuncture on each laboratory slip. This aids in the interpretation of the temporal pattern of elevations.
- If a qualitative immunoassay is to be done at the bedside, 1.5 ml of whole blood is obtained in a micropipette and placed in the sample well of the testing device. A red or purple color in the "read" zone indicates that 0.2 ng/ml or more cardiac troponin is present in the patient's blood.

After

- Apply pressure or a pressure dressing to the venipuncture site.

Abnormal findings

▲ **Increased levels**
   Myocardial injury
   Myocardial infarction

notes

T

tuberculin test (PPD skin test)

Type of test Skin

Normal findings Negative: reaction <5 mm

Test explanation

Although this test is used to detect tuberculosis (TB) infection, it is unable to indicate whether the infection is active or dormant. For this test, a *purified protein derivative (PPD)* of the tubercle bacillus is injected intradermally. If the patient is infected with TB (whether active or dormant), lymphocytes will recognize the PPD antigen and cause a local reaction; if the patient is not infected, no reaction will occur. If the test is negative and the physician strongly suspects TB, a "second-strength" PPD can be used. If this test is negative, the patient does not have TB. The PPD skin test usually becomes positive 6 weeks after infection. Once positive, the reaction usually persists for life.

The PPD test also can be used as part of a series of skin tests done to assess the immune system. If the immune system is nonfunctioning because of poor nutrition or chronic illness (e.g., neoplasia, infection), the PPD test will be negative despite the patient having had an active or a dormant TB infection. Other skin tests used to test immune function include *Candida*, mumps virus, and *Trichophyton* organisms to which most people in the United States have been exposed.

Contraindications

- Patients with known active TB
- Patients who have received *bacille Calmette-Guérin* (BCG) immunization against PPD because these patients will demonstrate a positive reaction to the PPD vaccination even though they have never had TB infection

Procedure and patient care

Before

- Assess the patient for previous history of TB. Report a positive history to the physician.
- Evaluate the patient's history for previous PPD results and BCG immunization.

During

- Prepare the patient's forearm with alcohol and allow it to dry.
- Intradermally inject the PPD. A skin wheal will occur.
- Circle the area with indelible ink.
- Record the time at which the PPD was injected.

After

- Read the results in 48 to 72 hours.
- Examine the test site for induration (hardening). Measure the area of induration (not redness) in millimeters.
- If the test is positive, ensure that the physician is notified and the patient treated appropriately.
- If the test is positive, check the patient's arm 4 to 5 days after the test to be certain that a severe skin reaction has not occurred.

Abnormal findings

Positive results
TB infection
Nontuberculous mycobacteria infections

Negative result
Possible immunoincompetence

notes

T

TUMOR MARKERS

prostate-specific antigen (PSA)
CA 27.29 and CA 15-3 tumor markers (Cancer antigen 15-3)
CA 19-9 tumor marker (Cancer antigen 19-9)
CA-125 tumor marker (Cancer antigen-125)
Carcinoembryonic antigen (CEA)

Type of test Blood

Normal findings

PSA: <4 ng/ml
CA 27.29: <38 U/ml
CA 15-3: <22 U/ml
CA 19-9: <37 U/ml
CA-125: 0-35 U/ml
CEA: <5 ng/ml or 0-2.5 μg/L (SI units)

Test explanation

Tumor markers are used to assist in the diagnosis of various cancers. Some are used to identify cancers in the preclinical state. They can be used to indicate tumor burden at the time of initial diagnosis. The higher the serum levels, the greater the tumor burden. They are used to determine adequacy of treatment. A drastic reduction to normal in the tumor marker is expected with complete eradication of tumor. Tumor markers are used in post-treatment surveillance of cancers. A rapid rise in marker levels may be associated with a recurrent or progressive tumor growth. The markers are somewhat specific for certain cancers and are discussed separately.

PSA

PSA can be detected in all males. However, its level is greatly increased in patients with prostatic cancer. PSA assay is a sensitive test for identifying prostate cancer and monitoring its response to therapy.

Prostate-specific antigen is more sensitive and specific than other prostatic tumor markers such as prostatic acid phosphatase. Also, PSA is more accurate than PAP in monitoring response and recurrence of tumor after therapy.

PSA (and PAP) levels also may be minimally elevated in patients with benign prostatic hypertrophy (BPH) and prostatitis. PSA levels greater than 10 ng/ml indicate a high probability for prostate cancer. Lower values may be compatible with BPH or early prostate cancer. Several formulas have been created to partially correct for BPH, which normally occurs in elderly men (e.g., predicted PSA = 0.12 × gland volume [in cubic centimeters] as determined by ultrasound). A rising PSA would also indicate cancer rather than BPH. PSA has been recommended for routine use in screening men over 50 years of age. When combined with direct digital rectal examination, it can detect 90% of prostate cancers.

CA 15-3 and CA 27.29

The CA 15-3 and CA 27.29 antigens are used for staging breast cancer and monitoring its treatment. CA 15-3 or CA 27.29 levels are high in less than 50% of patients whose presentation is a localized breast cancer or who have a small tumor burden. Of patients with metastatic breast cancer, however, 80% do have elevated CA 15-3 levels, and 65% have elevated CA 27.29 levels; therefore the usefulness of these antigen tests as a screening technique in early breast cancers (the most common cancer of women) is quite limited. Benign breast disease and nonbreast malignancies (such as lung, pancreas, ovary, and prostate) also can cause elevation of these antigen levels.

CA 19-9

CA 19-9 antigen is a tumor marker used in diagnosis and monitoring treatment of patients with pancreatic or hepatobiliary cancer. CA 19-9 is a carbohydrate antigen that exists on the surface of cancer cells. CA 19-9 levels may not be elevated in all patients with pancreatic carcinoma. Approximately 70% of patients with pancreatic carcinoma and 65% of patients with hepatobiliary cancer have elevated levels.

Mildly elevated CA 19-9 levels may exist in patients with gastric cancer, colorectal cancer, hepatoma, or nongastrointestinal malignancies. Patients who have pancreatitis, gallstones, cirrhosis, inflammatory bowel disease, or cystic fibrosis also can have minimally elevated levels of CA 19-9. Because of its lack of sensitivity and specificity, CA 19-9 is not effective in screening for pancreaticobiliary tumors in the general population.

CA-125

CA-125 is an extremely accurate marker for nonmucinous epithelial tumors of the ovary. It is elevated in over 80% of women with ovarian cancer. This tumor marker has a high degree of sensitivity and specificity for ovarian cancer and has been of great benefit to clinicians.

The CA-125 serum tumor marker is also used to determine a patient's response to therapy. Also CA-125 tumor markers can predict whether or not a second-look (repeat) diagnostic laparotomy will be positive. A precipitous fall in CA-125 after two courses of chemotherapy is an accurate predictor of a complete response to chemotherapy and is used as a good prognostic sign.

CA-125 is not an effective screening test for the asymptomatic general public because of its lack of specificity. It is used in a "high-risk" population of women who have a strong family history of ovarian cancer. Elevated levels in the general population indicate that either benign or malignant disease is present in 95% of patients.

Other tumors and benign processes can cause elevated CA-125 levels as well. Diseases that affect the peritoneum such as cirrhosis, pancreatitis, peritonitis, endometriosis, and pelvic inflammatory disease can create elevated levels of CA-125. Other malignancies occurring in the female genital tract, pancreas, colon, lung, and breast can also be associated with elevated levels of this protein. Of the normal population, 1% to 2% have CA-125 levels in excess of 35 U/mL.

CEA

CEA exists in the bloodstream of adults who have colorectal tumors. This protein is also found in patients who have a variety of carcinomas (e.g., breast, pancreatic, gastric, hepatobiliary), sarcomas, and even many benign diseases (e.g., ulcerative colitis, diverticulitis, cirrhosis). It is important to note that many patients with advanced breast or gastrointestinal tumors may not have elevated CEA levels.

Because the CEA level can be elevated in both benign and malignant diseases, it is not considered to be a specific test for colorectal cancer. As a result, CEA is not a reliable screening test for the detection of colorectal cancer in the general population.

CEA can also be detected in body fluids other than blood. Its presence in those fluids indicates metastasis. This antigen is commonly measured in peritoneal fluid or chest effusions. An elevated CEA in these fluids indicates metastasis to the peritoneum or pleura, respectively.

Interfering factors

PSA

- Rectal examinations, known to falsely elevate PAP levels, may also minimally elevate PSA levels.
- Prostatic manipulation by biopsy or transurethral resection of the prostate (TURP) may elevate the PSA levels. The blood test should be done before the surgery or 6 weeks afterwards.

CA-125

- The first trimester of pregnancy and normal menstruation may be associated with mild elevations of CA-125 levels.

CEA

- Chronic smokers have elevated CEA levels.

Procedure and patient care

Before

- Tell the patient that no fasting is required.

During

- Collect approximately 5 ml of blood in a red-top tube.

After

- Apply pressure to the venipuncture site.

Abnormal findings

▲ **Increased PSA levels**
  Prostate cancer
  Benign prostatic hypertrophy
  Prostatitis

▲ **Increased CA 27.29 or CA 15-3 levels**
  Metastatic breast cancer

▲ **Increased CA 19-9 levels**
  Pancreatic carcinoma
  Hepatobiliary carcinoma
  Pancreatitis
  Cholecystitis
  Cirrhosis
  GI malignancy
  Gallstones
  Cystic fibrosis

T

▲ **Increased CA-125 levels**

Malignant disorders
Cancer of the ovary
Cancer of the pancreas
Cancer of the nonovarian female genital tract
Cancer of the breast
Cancer of the colon
Cancer of the lung
Lymphoma
Peritoneal carcinomatosis
Benign disorders
Cirrhosis
Peritonitis
Pregnancy
Endometriosis
Pancreatitis
Pelvic inflammatory disease

▲ **Increased CEA levels**
Cancer (gastrointestinal, breast, lung, pancreatic, hepatobiliary)
Inflammation (colitis, cholecystitis, pancreatitis, diverticulitis)
Cirrhosis

notes

UPPER GASTROINTESTINAL RADIOGRAPHY

upper gastrointestinal x-ray study (Upper GI series, UGI)

barium swallow

Type of test X-ray with contrast dye

Normal findings Normal size, contour, patency, filling, positioning, and transit of barium through the esophagus, stomach, and upper duodenum

Test explanation

The upper GI study consists of a series of x-ray films of the lower esophagus, stomach, and duodenum, usually using barium sulfate as the contrast medium. The barium swallow is a more thorough examination of the esophagus than that provided by most upper GI series.

Defects in normal filling and narrowing of the barium column in the esophagus indicate tumor, strictures, or extrinsic compression from extraesophageal tumors or an abnormally enlarged heart and great vessels. Varices also can be seen as serpiginous, linear-filling defects. Anatomic abnormalities such as hiatal hernia, Shatzski's rings, and diverticula (Zenker's or epiphrenic) can be seen as well. Esophageal muscular abnormalities such as achalasia, as well as diffuse esophageal spasm, can be easily detected by a barium swallow.

Ulcerations, tumors, inflammations, or anatomic malpositions involving the stomach or duodenum can be seen. Obstruction of the upper GI tract is also easily detected.

In patients with gastroesophageal reflux, the radiologist may identify reflux of the barium from the stomach back into the esophagus. The small intestine can then be studied by a small bowel follow-through.

Contraindications

- Patients with evidence of bowel obstruction. Barium may create a stonelike impaction.
- Patients with a perforated viscus. Usually, when perforation is suspected, diatrizoate (Gastrografin), a water-soluble contrast medium, is used.

U

Potential complications

- Aspiration of barium
- Constipation or partial bowel obstruction caused by inspissated barium in the small bowel or colon

Interfering factors

- Previously administered barium may block visualization of the upper GI tract.
- Food and fluid in the stomach may give the false impression of a filling defect (tumor) within the stomach.

Procedure and patient care

Before

- Instruct the patient to abstain from eating for at least 8 hours before the test. Usually keep the patient NPO after midnight on the day of the test.
- Assess the patient's ability to swallow. If the patient tends to aspirate, inform the radiologist.

During

- Note the following procedural steps:
  1. The patient is asked to drink approximately 16 ounces of barium sulfate. This is a chalky substance usually suspended in milkshake form and drunk through a straw. Usually the drink is flavored to increase palatability.
  2. As the patient drinks the contrast through a straw, the x-ray table is tilted to the near-erect position.
  3. The patient is asked to roll into various positions so that the entire upper GI tract can be adequately visualized.
  4. The flow of barium is followed through the lower esophagus, stomach, and duodenum.
  5. Films are taken at the discretion of the radiologist observing the flow of barium fluoroscopically.
- In an *air-contrast upper GI study,* the patient is asked to swallow rapidly carbonated powder. This creates carbon dioxide in the stomach, providing air contrast to the barium within the upper GI tract.

After

- Inform the patient that, if Gastrografin was used, he or she may have significant diarrhea. Gastrografin is an osmotic cathartic.
- Instruct the patient to use a cathartic (e.g., milk of magnesia) if barium sulfate was used as the contrast medium.

Water absorption may cause the barium to harden and create a fecal impaction if catharsis is not carried out.

- Instruct the patient to watch his or her stools to ensure that all of the barium has been removed. The stools should return to normal color after completely expelling the barium, which may take as much as a day and a half.

Abnormal findings

Esophageal strictures/rings
Achalasia/chalasia
Esophageal motility disorders
Esophageal cancer
Esophageal varices
Hiatal hernia
Esophageal diverticula
Gastric cancer
Gastric inflammatory disease (e.g., Ménétrier's disease)
Benign gastric tumor (e.g., leiomyoma)
Extrinsic compression by pancreatic pseudocysts, cysts, pancreatic tumors, or hepatomegaly
Perforation of the esophagus, stomach, or duodenum
Congenital abnormalities (e.g., duodenal web, pancreatic rest, malrotation syndrome)
Gastric ulcer (benign and malignant)
Gastritis
Duodenal ulcer
Duodenal cancer
Duodenal diverticulum

notes

U

urea nitrogen blood test (Blood urea nitrogen [BUN], Serum urea nitrogen)

Type of test Blood

Normal findings
Adult: 10-20 mg/dl or 3.6-7.1 mmol/L (SI units)
Elderly: may be slightly higher
Child: 5-18 mg/dl
Infant: 5-18 mg/dl
Newborn: 3-12 mg/dl
Cord: 21-40 mg/dl

Possible critical values >100 mg/dl (indicates serious impairment of renal function)

Test explanation
BUN is directly related to the metabolic function of the liver and the excretory function of the kidney. It serves as an index of the function of these organs. Patients who have elevated BUN levels are said to have azotemia.

Nearly all renal diseases cause an inadequate excretion of urea, which causes the blood concentration to rise above normal. If the disease is unilateral, however, the unaffected kidney can compensate for the diseased kidney, and the BUN may not become elevated. The BUN also increases in conditions other than primary renal disease. For example, when excess amounts of protein are available for hepatic catabolism (from a high-protein diet or gastrointestinal [GI] bleeding), large quantities of urea are made. BUN levels also may vary according to the state of hydration, with increased levels seen in dehydration and decreased levels seen in overhydration. Finally, one must be aware that the synthesis of urea depends on the liver. Patients with severe primary liver disease will have a decreased BUN. With combined liver and renal disease (as in hepatorenal syndrome), the BUN can be normal not because renal excretory function is good but because poor hepatic functioning has resulted in decreased formation of urea.

The BUN is interpreted in conjunction with the creatinine test (see p. 98). These tests are referred to as *renal function studies.*

Procedure and patient care

Before
- Tell the patient that no fasting is required.

During
- Collect approximately 5 ml of blood in a red-top tube.

After
- Apply pressure or a pressure dressing to the venipuncture site.

Abnormal findings

▲ **Increased levels**

Prerenal causes
Hypovolemia
Shock
Burns
Dehydration
Congestive heart failure
Myocardial infarction
GI bleeding
Excessive protein ingestion
Alimentary tube feeding
Excessive protein catabolism
Starvation
Sepsis
Renal causes
Renal disease (e.g., glomerulonephritis, pyelonephritis, acute tubular necrosis)
Renal failure
Nephrotoxic drugs
Postrenal azotemia
Ureteral obstruction
Bladder outlet obstruction

▼ **Decreased levels**
Liver failure
Overhydration caused by fluid overload or SIADH syndrome
Negative nitrogen balance (e.g., malnutrition or malabsorption)
Pregnancy
Nephrotic syndrome

U

uric acid, blood

Type of test Blood

Normal findings

Blood
Adult
Male: 2.1-8.5 mg/dl or 0.15-0.48 mmol/L
Female: 2-6.6 mg/dl or 0.09-0.36 mmol/L
Elderly: values may be slightly increased
Child: 2.5-5.5 mg/dl or 0.12-0.32 mmol/L
Newborn: 2-6.2 mg/dl

Possible critical values Blood >12 mg/dl

Test explanation

Uric acid is a nitrogenous compound that is a product of purine (a deoxyribonucleic acid [DNA] building block) catabolism. When uric acid levels are elevated (hyperuricemia), the patient may have gout. Causes of hyperuricemia can be overproduction or decreased excretion of uric acid (e.g., kidney failure). Overproduction of uric acid may occur in patients with a catabolic enzyme deficiency that stimulates purine metabolism or in patients with cancer in whom purine and DNA turnover is great. Other causes of hyperuricemia may include alcoholism, leukemias, metastatic cancer, multiple myeloma, hyperlipoproteinemia, diabetes mellitus, renal failure, stress, lead poisoning, and dehydration caused by diuretic therapy. Ketoacids (as occur in diabetic or alcoholic ketoacidosis) may compete with uric acid for tubular excretion and may cause decreased uric acid excretion. Many causes of hyperuricemia are undefined and therefore labeled as *idiopathic*.

Elevated uric acid in the urine is called uricosuria. Uric acid can become supersaturated in the urine and crystallize to form kidney stones that can block the renal system. Uric acid is less well saturated in an acidic urine. As the urine pH rises, more uric acid can exist without crystallization and stone formation. Therefore, when a person is known to have high uric acid in the urine, the urine can be alkalinized by ingestion of a strong base to prevent stone formation.

Procedure and patient care

Before
- Follow the institution's requirements regarding fasting. (Some recommend that the patient fast.)

During
- Collect approximately 5 to 7 ml of venous blood in a red-top tube.

After
- Apply pressure to the venipuncture site.

Abnormal findings

▲ **Increased blood levels (hyperuricemia)**
Gout
Increased ingestion of purines
Genetic inborn error in purine metabolism
Metastatic cancer
Multiple myeloma
Leukemias
Cancer chemotherapy
Hemolysis
Rhabdomyolysis (e.g., heavy exercise, burns, crush injury, epileptic seizure, or myocardial infarction)
Chronic renal disease
Acidosis (ketotic or lactic)
Hypothyroidism
Toxemia of pregnancy
Hyperlipoproteinemia
Alcoholism
Shock or chronic blood volume depletion states
Idiopathic

▼ **Decreased blood levels**
Wilson's disease
Fanconi syndrome
Lead poisoning
Yellow atrophy of the liver

U

urinalysis (UA)

Type of test   Urine

Normal findings

Appearance: clear
Color: amber yellow
Odor: aromatic
pH: 4.6-8.0 (average 6.0)
Protein
   None or up to 8 mg/dl
   50-80 mg/dl (at rest)
   <250 mg/dl (exercise)
Specific gravity
   Adult: 1.005-1.030 (usually 1.010-1.025)
   Elderly: values decrease with age
   Newborn: 1.001-1.020
Leukocyte esterase: negative
Nitrites: negative
Ketones: negative
Crystals: negative
Casts: none present
Glucose (see urine glucose discussion, p. 142)
   Brand new specimen: negative
   24-hour specimen: <0.5 g/dl or <70 mmol/day (SI units)
White blood cells (WBCs): 0-4 per low-power field
WBC casts: negative
Red blood cells (RBCs): up to 2 per low-power field
RBC casts: none

Test explanation

  A total urinalysis involves multiple routine tests on a urine specimen. This specimen is not necessarily a clean-catch specimen. Routinely a urinalysis includes remarks about the color, appearance, and odor of the urine. The pH is determined. The urine is tested for the presence of proteins, glucose, ketones, blood, and leukocyte esterase. The urine is examined microscopically for RBCs, WBCs, casts, crystals, and bacteria.

  Examination of the urine sediment provides a significant amount of information about the urinary system. The test is done on a centrifuged urinary sediment.

Appearance and color

Urine appearance and color are noted as part of routine urinalysis. The appearance of a normal urine specimen should be clear. Cloudy urine may be caused by the presence of pus, RBCs, or bacteria; however, normal urine also may be cloudy because of ingestion of certain foods (e.g., large amounts of fat, ureates, or phosphates). The color of urine ranges from pale yellow to amber. The color indicates the concentration of the urine. Dilute urine is straw colored, and concentrated urine is deep amber.

Abnormally colored urine may result from a pathologic condition or the ingestion of certain foods or medicines. Many frequently used drugs also may affect urine color.

Odor

Determination of urine odor is a part of routine urinalysis. The aromatic odor of fresh, normal urine is caused by the presence of volatile acids. Urine of patients with diabetic ketoacidosis has the strong, sweet smell of acetone. In patients with a urinary tract infection, the urine may have a very foul odor. Patients with a fecal odor to their urine may have an enterobladder fistula.

pH

The analysis of the pH of a freshly voided urine specimen indicates the acid-base balance of the patient. An alkaline pH is obtained in a patient with alkalemia. Also, bacteria, urinary tract infection, or a diet high in citrus fruits or vegetables may cause an increased urine pH. Certain medications (e.g., streptomycin, neomycin, kanamycin) are effective in treating urinary tract infections when the urine is alkaline. Acidic urine is generally obtained in patients with acidemia, which can result from metabolic or respiratory acidosis, starvation, dehydration, or a diet high in meat products or cranberries.

The urine pH is useful in identifying crystals in the urine and determining the predisposition to form a given type of stone. Acidic urine is associated with xanthine, cystine, uric acid, and calcium oxalate stones. To treat or prevent these urinary calculi, urine should be kept alkaline. Alkaline urine is associated with calcium carbonate, calcium phosphate, and magnesium phosphate stones; for these stones urine should be kept acidic.

Protein

Evaluation of protein is a sensitive indicator of kidney function. Normally protein is not present in the urine. The combination of proteinuria and edema is known as the nephrotic syndrome.

Proteinuria is probably the most important indicator of renal disease. The urine of all pregnant women is routinely checked for proteinuria, which can be an indicator of preeclampsia. In addition to screening for nephrotic syndrome, urinary protein also screens for complications of diabetes mellitus, glomerulonephritis, amyloidosis, and multiple myeloma.

Glucose

See discussion on p. 142.

Specific gravity

The specific gravity is a measure of the concentration of particles, including wastes and electrolytes, in the urine. A high specific gravity indicates a concentrated urine; a low specific gravity indicates dilute urine.

The specific gravity is used to evaluate the concentrating and excretory power of the kidney. Renal disease tends to diminish the concentrating capability of the kidney. As a result, chronic renal diseases are associated with a low specific gravity. The specific gravity is also a measurement of the hydration status of the patient. An overhydrated patient will have a more dilute urine with a lower specific gravity. The specific gravity of the urine in a dehydrated patient can be expected to be abnormally high.

Leukocyte esterase (WBC esterase)

Leukocyte (WBC) esterase is a screening test used to detect leukocytes in the urine. When positive, this test indicates a urinary tract infection.

Nitrites

Like the leukocyte esterase, the nitrite test is a screening test for the identification of urinary tract infections.

Ketones

Normally no ketones are present in the urine; however, a patient with poorly controlled diabetes who is hyperglycemic may have massive fatty acid catabolism. This test for ketonuria is also important in evaluating ketoacidosis associated with alcoholism, fasting, starvation, high-protein diets, and isopropanol ingestion. Ketonuria may occur with acute febrile illnesses, especially in infants and children.

Crystals

Crystals found in the urinary sediment on microscopic examination indicate that renal stone formulation is imminent, if not already present.

Casts

Casts are clumps of materials or cells. They are formed in the renal distal and collecting tubules where the material is maximally concentrated. Casts are most usually associated with some degree of proteinuria and stasis within the renal tubules. There are several kinds of casts: hyaline and cellular.

Hyaline casts are conglomerations of protein and indicate proteinuria. A few hyaline casts are normally found.

Cellular casts, conglomerations of degenerated cells, are described in the following paragraphs.

Granular casts result from the disintegration of cellular material into granular particles within a WBC or epithelial cell cast.

Waxy casts may be cell casts, hyaline casts, or renal failure casts.

Large numbers of epithelial cells are abnormal and can conglomerate into *tubular (epithelial) casts.* These are most suggestive of glomerulonephritis.

Normally few WBCs are found in the urine sediment on microscopic examination. The presence of five or more WBCs in the urine indicates a urinary tract infection involving the bladder, kidney, or both. *WBC casts* are most frequently found in patients with infections within the kidney, such as acute pyelonephritis.

Any disruption in the blood-urine barrier whether at the glomerular, tubular, ureteral, or bladder level will cause RBCs to enter the urine. The bleeding can be microscopic or gross hematuria. *RBC casts* suggest glomerulonephritis. RBC casts are also seen in patients with acute necrosis, pyelonephritis, renal trauma, or renal tumor.

Interfering factors

- Urine color darkens with prolonged standing.
- When urine stands for a long time and begins to decompose, it has an ammonia-like smell.
- The urine pH becomes alkaline on standing because of the action of urea-splitting bacteria, producing ammonia.
- The urine pH of an uncovered specimen will become alkaline because carbon dioxide will vaporize from the urine and into the air.
- Urine contaminated with vaginal secretions may cause proteinuria.

- Recent use of radiographic dyes in the urine increases specific gravity.
- False-positive leukocyte esterase results may occur in specimens contaminated with vaginal secretions.
- Vaginal discharge may contaminate the urine specimen and factitiously cause WBCs in the urine.
- Strenuous physical exercise may cause RBC casts. Traumatic urethral catheterization may cause RBCs in the urine.
- Drugs that may affect urine color include antibiotics and vitamins.
- Drugs that may cause acidic urine include ammonium chloride, chlorothiazide diuretics, and methenamine mandelate.
- Drugs that may cause alkaline urine include acetazolamide, potassium citrate, and sodium bicarbonate.
- Drugs that may cause *increased* specific gravity include dextran and sucrose.

Procedure and patient care

Before

- Explain the procedure to the patient.

During

- Collect a fresh urine specimen in a urine container.
- If the urine specimen contains vaginal discharge or bleeding, a clean-catch or midstream specimen will be needed (see urine culture, p. 103).
- For ketones a test can be performed immediately after collection by placing a drop of urine on an Acetest tablet. If acetone is present, shades of lavender will appear at the designated time.
- To test for ketones with a Ketostix, dip the reagent into the urine specimen and remove it. Read the strip in 15 seconds by comparing it with the color chart.

After

- Transport the urine specimen to the laboratory promptly.
- If the specimen cannot be processed immediately, refrigerate it.
- Casts will break up as urine is allowed to sit. Urine examinations for casts should be performed on fresh specimens.

Abnormal findings

Appearance and color

Bacteria
Pus
Red blood cells
Certain foods (e.g., beets, carrots)
Drug therapy
Pathologic conditions (e.g., bleeding from the kidney)

Dehydration
Overhydration
Diabetes insipidus
Fever
Excessive sweating
Jaundice

Odor

Infection
Ketonuria
Urinary tract infection
Rectal fistula

Maple sugar urine disease
Phenylketonuria
Hepatic failure

pH

▲ **Increased levels**
   Respiratory alkalosis
   Metabolic alkalosis
   Urea-splitting bacteria
   Vegetarian diet
   Renal failure with inability to form ammonia
   Gastric suction
   Vomiting
   Diuretic therapy
   Renal tubular acidosis
   Urinary tract infection

▼ **Decreased levels**
   Metabolic acidosis
   Diabetes mellitus
   Diarrhea
   Starvation
   Respiratory acidosis
   Emphysema
   Sleep
   Pyrexia

Protein

▲ **Increased levels**
   Nephrotic syndrome
   Diabetes mellitus
   Multiple myeloma
   Preeclampsia
   Glomerulonephritis
   Congestive heart failure
   Malignant hypertension
   Polycystic disease
   Diabetic glomerulosclerosis

▼ **Decreased levels**
   Amyloidosis
   Lupus erythematosus
   Goodpasture syndrome
   Renal vein thrombosis
   Heavy-metal poisoning
   Galactosemia
   Bacterial pyelonephritis
   Nephrotoxic drug therapy
   Bladder tumor

U

Specific gravity

▲ **Increased levels**
Dehydration
Pituitary tumor or trauma
that causes syndrome of
inappropriate release of
excessive antidiuretic
hormone (SIADH)
Decrease in renal blood
flow (as in heart failure,
renal artery stenosis, or
hypotension)
Glycosuria and proteinuria
Water restriction
Fever
Excessive sweating
Vomiting
Diarrhea
X-ray contrast dye

▼ **Decreased levels**
Overhydration
Diabetes insipidus
Renal failure
Diuresis
Hypothermia
Glomerulonephritis
Pyelonephritis

Leukocyte esterase

Possible urinary tract infection

Nitrites

Possible urinary tract infection

Ketones

Uncontrolled diabetes mellitus
Starvation
Excessive aspirin ingestion
Ketoacidosis of alcoholism
Febrile illnesses in infants and
children
Weight reduction diets

Following anesthesia
Prolonged vomiting
Anorexia
Fasting
High-protein diets
Isopropanol ingestion
Dehydration

Crystals

Renal stone formation
Drug therapy
Urinary tract infection

Granular casts

Acute tubular necrosis
Urinary tract infection
Glomerulonephritis
Pyelonephritis
Nephrosclerosis

Chronic lead poisoning
Reaction after exercise
Stress
Renal transplant rejection

Fatty casts

Nephrotic syndrome
Diabetic nephropathy

Glomerulonephritis
Chronic renal disease

Epithelial casts

Glomerulonephritis
Eclampsia
Heavy-metal poisoning

Ethylene glycol intoxication
Acute renal allograft rejection

Waxy casts

Chronic renal disease
Chronic renal failure
Diabetic nephropathy
Malignant hypertension

Glomerulonephritis
Renal transplant rejection
Nephrotic syndrome

Hyaline casts

Proteinuria
Fever
Strenuous exercise
Stress

Glomerulonephritis
Pyelonephritis
Congestive heart failure
Chronic renal failure

Red blood cells and casts

▲ **Increased RBC levels**
   Glomerulonephritis
   Interstitial nephritis
   Acute tubular necrosis
   Pyelonephritis
   Renal trauma
   Renal tumor
   Renal stones
   Cystitis
   Prostatitis
   Traumatic bladder
      catheterization

▲ **Increased RBC cast levels**
   Glomerulonephritis
   Subacute bacterial endocarditis
   Renal infarct
   Goodpasture syndrome
   Vasculitis
   Sickle cell anemia
   Malignant hypertension
   Systemic lupus erythematosus

White blood cells and casts

▲ **Increased WBC levels**
   Bacterial infection in the
      urinary tract

▲ **Increased WBC cast levels**
   Acute pyelonephritis
   Glomerulonephritis
   Lupus nephritis

U

white blood cell count and differential count (WBC and differential, Leukocyte count, Neutrophil count, Lymphocyte count, Monocyte count, Eosinophil count, Basophil count)

Type of test Blood

Normal findings

Total WBCs

Adult/child >2 years: 5000-10,000/mm^3 or 5-10 × 10^9/L (SI units)

Child ≤2 years: 6200-17,000/mm^3

Newborn: 9000-30,000/mm^3

Differential count

	(%)	Absolute (per mm^3)
Neutrophils	55 to 70	2500-8000
Lymphocytes	20 to 40	1000-4000
Monocytes	2 to 8	100-700
Eosinophils	1 to 4	50-500
Basophils	0.5 to 1	25-100

Possible critical values WBCs <2500 or >30,000/mm^3

Test explanation

The WBC count has two components. The first is a count of the total number of WBCs (leukocytes) in 1 mm^3 of peripheral venous blood. The other component, the differential count, measures the percentage of each type of leukocyte present in the same specimen. Neutrophils and lymphocytes make up 75% to 90% of the total leukocytes. An increased total WBC count (leukocytosis: WBC >10,000) usually indicates infection, inflammation, tissue necrosis, or leukemic neoplasia. Trauma or stress, either emotional or physical, may increase the WBC count. A decreased total WBC count (leukopenia: WBC <4,000) occurs in many forms of bone marrow failure (e.g., following antineoplastic chemotherapy or radiation therapy, marrow infiltrative diseases, overwhelming infections, dietary deficiencies, and autoimmune diseases).

White blood cells are divided into granulocytes and nongranulocytes. Granulocytes include neutrophils, basophils, and eosinophils. Granulocytes have multilobed nuclei and are sometimes referred to as polymorphonuclear leukocytes (PMNs or "polys").

Neutrophils are the most common PMN. Acute bacterial infections and trauma stimulate neutrophil production, resulting in an increased WBC count. Often, when neutrophil production is significantly stimulated, early immature forms of neutrophils enter the circulation. These immature forms are called *band* or *stab* cells. This occurrence, referred to as a "shift to the left" in WBC production, is indicative of an ongoing acute bacterial infection.

Basophils (also called mast cells), and especially *eosinophils,* are involved in an allergic reaction. Parasitic infestations also are capable of stimulating the production of these cells.

Nongranulocytes (agranulocytes) include lymphocytes and monocytes (the count also includes histiocytes).

Lymphocytes are divided into two types: T cells and B cells. T cells are involved with cellular immunity (e.g., "killer cells"). B cells participate in humoral immunity (i.e., antibody production).

Monocytes are phagocytic cells capable of fighting bacteria in a way very similar to that of neutrophils.

The WBC and differential count are routinely measured as part of the *complete blood count (CBC).* Serial WBC counts and differential counts have both diagnostic and prognostic value. For example, a persistent increase in the WBC count may indicate a worsening of an infectious process (e.g., appendicitis). A dramatic decrease in the WBC count below the normal range may indicate marrow failure. In patients receiving chemotherapy, a reduced WBC count may delay further chemotherapy.

Interfering factors

- Patients who have had a splenectomy have a persistent, mild elevation of WBC counts.

Procedure and patient care

Before
- Tell the patient that no fasting is required.

During
- Collect approximately 5 to 7 ml of venous blood in a lavender-top tube.

After

- Apply pressure to the venipuncture site.

Abnormal findings

▲ **Increased WBC count (leukocytosis)**
Infection
Leukemic neoplasia
Trauma
Stress
Tissue necrosis
Inflammation

▼ **Decreased WBC count (leukopenia)**
Drug toxicity (e.g., chloramphenicol)
Bone marrow failure
Overwhelming infections
Dietary deficiency
Autoimmune disease
Bone marrow infiltration (e.g., myelofibrosis)
Congenital marrow aplasia

▲▼ **Increased/decreased differential count**
See Table 4.

notes

TABLE 4 Causes for abnormalities in the WBC differential count

Type of WBC	Elevated	Decreased
Neutrophils	*Neutrophilia* Physical or emotional stress Acute suppurative infection Myelocytic leukemia Trauma Cushing's syndrome Inflammatory disorders (e.g., rheumatic fever, thyroiditis, rheumatoid arthritis) Metabolic disorders (e.g., ketoacidosis, gout, eclampsia)	*Neutropenia* Aplastic anemia Dietary deficiency Overwhelming bacterial infection (especially in the elderly) Viral infections (e.g., hepatitis, influenza, measles) Radiation therapy Addison's disease Drug therapy: myelotoxic drugs (as in chemotherapy)
Lymphocytes	*Lymphocytosis* Chronic bacterial infection Viral infection (e.g., mumps, rubella) Lymphocytic leukemia Multiple myeloma Infectious mononucleosis Radiation Infectious hepatitis	*Lymphocytopenia* Leukemia Sepsis Immunodeficiency diseases Lupus erythematosus Later stages of human immunodeficiency virus infection Drug therapy: adrenocorticosteroids, antineoplastics Radiation therapy

W

Continued

TABLE 4 Causes for abnormalities in the WBC differential count—cont'd

Type of WBC	Elevated	Decreased
Monocytes	*Monocytosis* Chronic inflammatory disorders Viral infections (e.g., infectious mononucleosis) Tuberculosis Chronic ulcerative colitis Parasites (e.g., malaria)	*Monocytopenia* Drug therapy: prednisone
Eosinophils	*Eosinophilia* Parasitic infections Allergic reactions Eczema Leukemia Autoimmune diseases	*Eosinopenia* Increased adrenosteroid production
Basophils	*Basophilia* Myeloproliferative disease (e.g., myelofibrosis, polycythemia rubra vera) Leukemia	*Basopenia* Acute allergic reactions Hyperthyroidism Stress reactions

Appendix A: Alphabetical list of tests

Appendix B: Abbreviations for diagnostic and laboratory tests

A	ABGs	Arterial blood gases
	AFP	Alpha-fetoprotein
	A/G ratio	Albumin/globulin ratio
	AIT	Agglutination inhibition test
	ALP	Alkaline phosphatase
	ALT	Alanine aminotransferase
	ANA	Antinuclear antibody
	APTT	Activated partial thromboplastin time
	AST	Aspartate aminotransferase
B	BE	Barium enema
	BMC	Bone mineral content
	BMD	Bone marrow density
	BRCA	Breast cancer
	BUN	Blood urea nitrogen
C	Ca	Calcium
	CC	Creatine clearance
	C&S	Culture and sensitivity
	CAT	Computerized axial tomography
	CBC	Complete blood count
	CEA	Carcinoembryonic antigen
	CK	Creatine kinase
	Cl	Chloride
	CO	Carbon monoxide
	CO_2	Carbon dioxide
	COHb	Carboxyhemoglobin test
	CPK, CP	Creatine phosphokinase
	CSF	Cerebrospinal fluid
	CST	Contraction stress test
	CT	Computed tomography
	CXR	Chest x-ray
D	DEXA	Dual-energy x-ray absorptiometry
	DMSA	Disodium monomethanearsonate renal scan
	DPA	Dual-photon absorptiometry
	DSA	Digital subtraction angiography
E	EBV	Epstein-Barr virus
	ECG, EKG	Electrocardiogram
	ECHO	Echocardiography
	EGD	Esophagogastroduodenoscopy

	EIA	Enzyme immunoassay
	ELISA	Enzyme-linked immunosorbent assay
	ER	Estrogen receptor
	ERCP	Endoscopic retrograde cholangiopancreatography
	ESR	Erythrocyte sedimentation rate
	EtOH	Ethanol, ethyl alcohol
	EUG	Excretory urography
F	FBS	Fasting blood sugar
	FDPs	Fibrin degradation products
	Fe	Iron
	FSH	Follicle-stimulating hormone
	FSPs	Fibrin split products
	FTA-ABS	Fluorescent treponemal antibody absorption test
	FT4	Thyroxin, free
G	GFR	Glomerular filtration rate
	GGT	Gamma-glutamyl transferase
	GGTP	Gamma-glutamyl transpeptidase
	GHb, GHB	Glycosylated hemoglobin
	GI series	Gastrointestinal series
	GTT	Glucose tolerance test
H	HAA	Hepatitis-associated antigen
	HAI	Hemagglutination inhibition
	Hb, Hgb	Hemoglobin
	HCG	Human chorionic gonadotropin
	HCO_3^-	Bicarbonate
	Hct	Hematocrit
	HDL	High-density lipoprotein
	H&H	Hemoglobin and hematocrit
	HIDA	Hepatic iminodiacetic acid
	HIV	Human immunodeficiency virus
	HTLV	Human T-cell lymphotrophic virus
I	Ig	Immunoglobulin
	INR	International normalization ratio
	IVP	Intravenous pyelography
	IVU, IUG	Intravenous urography
K	K	Potassium
	KS	Ketosteroid
	KUB	Kidney, ureter, and bladder x-ray study
L	LA	Latex agglutination
	LDH	Lactic dehydrogenase
	LDL	Low-density lipoprotein
	LFTs	Liver function tests

	LH	Luteinizing hormone
	LP	Lumbar puncture
	L/S ratio	Lecithin/sphingomyelin ratio
M	MCH	Mean corpuscular hemoglobin
	MCHC	Mean corpuscular hemoglobin concentration
	MCV	Mean corpuscular volume
	M/E ratio	Myeloid/erythroid ratio
	Mg	Magnesium
	MI	Maturation index
	MRI	Magnetic resonance imaging
N	Na	Sodium
	NMR	Nuclear magnetic resonance
	NST	Nonstress test
O	OB	Occult blood
	OCT	Oxytocin challenge test
	OGTT	Oral glucose tolerance test
P	P	Phosphorus
	PAB	Prealbumin
	PAP	Prostatic acid phosphatase
	P_{CO_2}	Partial pressure of carbon dioxide
	PFTs	Pulmonary function tests
	pH	Hydrogen ion concentration
	PKU	Phenylketonuria
	PMN	Polymorphonuclear
	P_{O_2}	Partial pressure of oxygen
	PO_4	Phosphate
	PPD	Purified protein derivative
	PPG	Postprandial glucose
	PSA	Prostate-specific antigen
	PT	Prothrombin time
	PTT	Partial thromboplastin time
R	RBC	Red blood cell
	RDW	Red cell distribution width
	RF	Rheumatoid factor
	RIA	Radioimmunoassay
S	SBF	Small bowel follow-through
	SGOT	Serum glutamic-oxaloacetic transaminase
	SGPT	Serum glutamic-pyruvic transaminase
	SPECT	Single-photon emission computed tomography
T	T3	Triiodothyronine
	T4	Thyroxine
	TBPA	Thyroxine-binding prealbumin
	TEE	Transesophageal echocardiography

	TGs	Trigylcerides
	TIBC	Total iron-binding capacity
	TRH	Thyrotropin-releasing hormone
	TTE	Transthoracic echocardiography
U	UA	Urinalysis
	UGI series	Upper gastrointestinal series
	US	Ultrasound
V	VDRL	Venereal Disease Research Laboratory
	VLDL	Very low–density lipoprotein
	VMA	Vanillylmandelic acid
	VPS	Ventilation/perfusion scanning
W	WBC	White blood cell (count)

Appendix C: Typical abbreviations and units of measurement

<	Less than
≤	Less than or equal to
>	Greater than
≥	Greater than or equal to
C	Celsius
cc	Cubic centimeter
cg	Centigram
cm	Centimeter
cm H_2O	Centimeter of water
cu	Cubic
dl	Deciliter (100 ml)
fmol	Femtomole
g	Gram
hr	Hour
IU	International unit
ImU	International milliunit
IμU	International microunit
K	Kilo
kg	Kilogram
L	Liter
m	Meter
m^2	Square meter
m^3	Cubic meter
mEq	Milliequivalent
mEq/L	Milliequivalent per liter
mg	Milligram
min	Minute
ml	Milliliter
mm	Millimeter
mm^3	Cubic millimeter
mM	Millimole
mm Hg	Millimeter of mercury
mm H_2O	Millimeter of water
mol	Mole
mmol	Millimole
mOsm	Milliosmole
mμ	Millimicron
mU	Milliunit

mV	Millivolt
ng	Nanogram
nm	Nanometer
nmol	Nanomole
Pa	Pascal
pg	Picogram (or micromicrogram)
pl	Picoliter
pm	Picometer
pmol	Picomole
sd	Standard deviation
sec	Second
SI units	International System of Units
μ	Micron
μ^3	Cubic micron
μg	Microgram
$I\mu U$	Microinternational unit
μl	Microliter
μm	Micrometer
μm^3	Cubic micrometer
μmol	Micromole
μU	Microunit
U	Unit
yr	Year

Bibliography

Barrick B, Vogel S: Application of laboratory diagnostics in HIV testing, *Nursing Clin North Am* 31(1):41-45, 1996.

Bates SE: Clinical applications of serum tumor markers, *Ann Intern Med* 115(8):623-634, 1991.

Braunwald E, editor: *Heart disease: a textbook of cardiovascular medicine,* ed 4, Philadelphia, 1992, WB Saunders.

Brooks MJ et al: The infectious etiology of peptic ulcer disease: diagnosis and implications for therapy, *Primary Care* 23(3):443-454, 1996.

Brunzel NA: *Fundamentals of urine and body fluid analysis,* Philadelphia, 1994, WB Saunders.

Casperson DS: Focus on oncology: prostatic specific antigen testing, *Urol Nurs* 11(1):31-34, 1992.

Cheney AM, Maquindang ML: Patient teaching for x-ray and other diagnostics, *RN* 56(4):54-56, 1993.

Coulter JS: Red blood cell distribution width and mean corpuscular volume: clinical applications, *Adv Clin Care* 6(6):13, 1991.

Creasy RK, Resnik R: *Maternal-fetal medicine: principles and practice,* ed 3, Philadelphia, 1994, WB Saunders.

Cupp MR, Oesterling JE: Prostate-specific antigen, digital rectal examination, and transrectal ultrasonography: their role in diagnosing early prostate cancer, *Mayo Clin Proc* 68:297-306, 1993.

De Veciana M et al: Postprandial versus preprandial blood glucose monitoring in women with gestational diabetes mellitus requiring insulin therapy, *N Engl J Med* 333(19):1237-1241, 1995.

Gregor CL: Antepartum fetal assessment techniques: an update for today's perinatal nurse, *J Perinatal Neonatal Nurs* 5(4):1-15, 1992.

Halfman-Francy M: Recognition and management of bleeding following cardiac surgery, *Crit Care Nurs Clin North Am* 3(4):675-689, 1991.

Henry JB: *Clinical diagnosis and laboratory management by laboratory methods,* ed 18, Philadelphia, 1991, WB Saunders.

Isselbacher KJ et al, editors: *Harrison's principles of internal medicine,* ed 13, New York, 1994, McGraw-Hill.

Kikuchi S et al: Serum anti-*Helicobacter pylori* antibody and gastric carcinoma among young adults, *Cancer* 75(12):2789-2792, 1995.

Koepke JA, editor: *Practical laboratory hematology,* New York, 1991, Churchill Livingstone.

Kuhlman JE: Oral and IV contrast-enhanced abdominal CT, *Appl Radiol* 21(10):20-21, 1992.

Lee GR et al, editors: *Wintrobe's clinical hematology,* ed 9, Philadelphia, 1993, Lea & Febiger.

Leitch AM et al: American Cancer Society guidelines for the early detection of breast cancer: update 1997, *Cancer* 47(3):150-153, 1997.

Lensing AW et al: A comparison of compression ultrasound with color Doppler ultrasound for diagnosis of symptomless postoperative deep vein thrombosis, *Arch Intern Med* 157(7):758-762, 1997.

Littrup PJ, Goodman AC, Mettlin CJ: The benefit and cost of prostate cancer early detection, *CA Cancer J Clin* 43(3):134-149, 1993.

McClatchey KD, editor: *Clinical laboratory medicine,* Baltimore, 1994, Williams & Wilkins.

Merva J: A closer look at the heart SAECG, *RN* 56(5):50-53, 1993.

Mettler FA et al: Benefits versus risks from mammography, *Cancer* 77(5):903-908, 1996.

Miller KE: Sexually transmitted diseases, *Primary Care* 24(1):179-193, 1997.

Pagana KD, Pagana TJ: *Mosby's diagnostic and laboratory test reference,* ed 4, St Louis, 1999, Mosby.

Pagana KD, Pagana TJ: *Mosby's manual of diagnostic and laboratory tests,* St Louis, 1998, Mosby.

Robie BH: Cardiovascular technology: noninvasive diagnosis of cardiovascular disease using ultrasound imaging, *J Cardiovasc Nurs* 6(2):36-42, 1992.

Sistrom C: Liver CT for cancer staging, *Appl Radiol* 21(6):19-24, 1992.

Thompson EJ: Transesophageal echocardiography: a new window on the heart and great vessels, *Crit Care Nurs* 13(10):55-56, 1993.

Thompson S: Ultrasonography: intraoperative diagnosis of choledocholithiasis, *AORN J* 51(4):983-985, 1990.

Wozniak-Petrofsky J: Prostate-specific antigen in prostate cancer, *J Urol Nurs* 12(3):104-105, 1992.

Wozniak-Petrofsky J: Basics of urodynamics, *J Urol Nurs* 12(2):434-463, 1993.

index